W9-DDI-419

AIDS

AIDS

Sigall K. Bell, MD,
Courtney L. McMickens, MD, MPH,
and
Kevin J. Selby, MD

Biographies of Disease
Julie K. Silver, MD, Series Editor

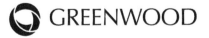

GREENWOOD

AN IMPRINT OF ABC-CLIO, LLC
Santa Barbara, California • Denver, Colorado • Oxford, England

Library of Congress Cataloging-in-Publication Data

Bell, Sigall K.
   AIDS / Sigall K. Bell, Kevin Selby and Courtney L. McMickens.
     p. cm. — (Biographies of disease)
   Includes bibliographical references and index.
   ISBN 978-0-313-37682-5 (hardback) — ISBN 978-0-313-37683-2 (ebook)
1. AIDS (Disease).   I. Selby, Kevin.   II. McMickens, Courtney L.   III. Title.

   RA643.8.B45   2011
   616.97'92—dc22   2011008460

ISBN: 978-0-313-37682-5
EISBN: 978-0-313-37683-2

15   14   13   12   11   1   2   3   4   5

This book is also available on the World Wide Web as an eBook.
Visit www.abc-clio.com for details.

Greenwood
An Imprint of ABC-CLIO, LLC

ABC-CLIO, LLC
130 Cremona Drive, P.O. Box 1911
Santa Barbara, California 93116–1911

This book is printed on acid-free paper ∞

Manufactured in the United States of America

Contents

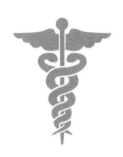

Series Foreword

Every disease has a story to tell: about how it started long ago and began to disable or even take the lives of its innocent victims, about the way it hurts us, and about how we are trying to stop it. In this Biographies of Disease series, the authors tell the stories of the diseases that we have come to know and dread.

The stories of these diseases have all of the components that make for great literature. There is incredible drama played out in real-life scenes from the past, present, and future. You'll read about how men and women of science stumbled trying to save the lives of those they aimed to protect. Turn the pages and you'll also learn about the amazing success of those who fought for health and won, often saving thousands of lives in the process.

If you don't want to be a health professional or research scientist now, when you finish this book you may think differently. The men and women in this book are heroes who often risked their own lives to save or improve ours. This is the biography of a disease, but it is also the story of real people who made incredible sacrifices to stop it in its tracks.

Julie K. Silver, MD
Assistant Professor, Harvard Medical School
Department of Physical Medicine and Rehabilitation

Preface

I magine the surprise and fear of doctors and patients faced with a new deadly illness of unknown cause. AIDS hit the medical community by storm, taking the lives of many people before it was recognized, identified, and named. Since that time, remarkable scientific discovery, dedicated care, activism, and courage have changed the shape of HIV—from a death sentence to the serious but manageable illness we know today.

Like few other illnesses, the AIDS story features a dramatic intersection of history, science, medicine, and society. In this book, we explore each of these perspectives, providing a broad understanding of HIV and AIDS. We start with a look back to the disease's early roots, exploring this new illness from the lens of patients and doctors who encountered it for the first time. Then we review the basic biology of HIV, including its viral structure and modes of replication. You will learn about the elegant way in which HIV—an incredibly simple yet effective infectious element—invades our immune cells. After discovering how HIV takes over our cellular machinery, we discuss its clever mechanisms for evading the immune system and eluding medications, and the great challenge it has posed to effective vaccine development. From there, we discuss the spread and impact of HIV, by studying the epidemiology of this global epidemic. We'll review risk factors associated with acquiring HIV and the way that HIV is transmitted, in addition to particular social or medical factors that facilitated transmission earlier in the epidemic. After that, we examine how the virus causing HIV was discovered and the effects this discovery had on diagnosis and treatment. This leads to a review of the now many effective medicines used to treat HIV, and their various mechanisms of actions. Also considered are the long-term consequences of HIV—the widespread effects on the body and the potential complications of the potent medications used to control the virus. This integrated view on HIV also allows us to discuss the cultural impact of this epidemic, and its profound effects on populations, family structure, economies, and politics. Finally, we look at the effect of the virus on a personal level—to understand the stigma once associated with this illness, and to celebrate the heroes and activists in the history of HIV. The book ends with a few personal accounts of what it is like to live with HIV, written by patients who wanted to share their story and a glimpse of what you can do to help.

As you embark on this journey ask yourself what biases or assumptions you have about AIDS and HIV and challenge yourself to think deeply and broadly about the issues presented. Along the way, we have provided "thought boxes" to encourage exploration of several themes or questions on your own or in discussion with others. The discovery of HIV has left a profound footprint on humanity for many reasons. We hope to enrich your views on the multiple domains in which it has left a historical impact, and perhaps pique your own interests in ways to get involved in HIV prevention or activism in the future.

Timeline

1981   First cases of pneumocystis pneumonia in IV drug users in New York City and Kaposi's sarcoma in Los Angeles.

1982   First use of the term "acquired immune deficiency syndrome," or AIDS.

1983   Documented heterosexual transmission. HIV (human immunodeficiency virus) proposed as the cause of AIDS by Luc Montagnier of France.

1984   Robert Gallo isolates HIV leading to the development of the Enzyme-Linked Immunosorbent Assay (ELISA) test to detect HIV antibodies. December 1 is the first World AIDS Day.

1985   Ryan White diagnosed with HIV test approved by the U.S. Food and Drug Administration (FDA).

1987   World Health Organization launches Global Programme on AIDS. Zidovudine (AZT) approved as first treatment for HIV.

1989   Dr. David Ho able to measure viral dynamics.

1990   Ryan White dies April 8 at age 18 of AIDS.

1991   Freddie Mercury, lead singer for Queen, dies 24 hours after announcing he has AIDS. Basketball star Magic Johnson announces that he is HIV positive.

1993   Early combination drug therapy in use, extending "AIDS-free" survival of HIV patients.

1995   Saquinavir, the first protease inhibitor, becomes available. Number of AIDS cases in the developed world begin to fall.

1996   Peak AIDS death rate in United States. The Joint United Nations Programme on HIV/AIDS (UNAIDS) created. Highly active antiretroviral therapy (HAART) launched resulting in a sharp decline in AIDS deaths.

2001   WHO and UNAIDS launch the 3x5 initiative. The Global Fund, to fight HIV/AIDS and malaria, launched.

2003   President Bush announces the President's Emergency Plan for AIDS Relief (PEPFAR).

2006   Luc Montagnier and Françoise Barre-Sinousi share the Nobel Prize for the isolation of HIV. U.S. Centers for Disease Control (CDC) recommends universal HIV testing. First single pill combination therapy taken once a day approved.

2007   With better data, UNAIDS lowers global prevalence estimate to 33 million people.

1

Historical Perspective: Where Did HIV Come From?

Kevin J. Selby, MD

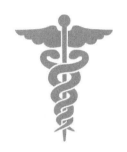

This chapter discusses the emergence of new diseases, the relationship of human illness to animal hosts, and the geographic origins of HIV. In this chapter we will address the following questions:

- What were the first described cases of HIV like?
- How was HIV discovered?
- How did we develop a test for HIV?
- What were the origins of HIV infection?
- What is SIV infection, and how is it related to HIV?

FIRST CASES

The first cases of HIV infection were terrifying medical mysteries. Early in 1981, previously healthy men in Los Angeles, San Francisco, and New York City started appearing in hospitals with an unusual infection in their lungs and a rare form of cancer on their skin. They were very sick, responded poorly to the treatments that were available, and baffled doctors across the country. Most of them deteriorated rapidly and nearly all of them died.

On June 5, 1981, the Centers for Disease Control (CDC), a government organization that tracks infectious diseases in the United States, published the first documentation of several cases that were later found to be HIV infection. Five men in Los Angeles between 29 and 36 years old had all been found to have pneumocystis pneumonia (PCP), and doctors thought that their infections might be related to each other. PCP is a rare form of pneumonia caused by a fungus that surrounds us everywhere in our environment, but it is usually easily neutralized by our immune system. The only people prior to this time who got PCP were people with severe problems with their immune systems and patients taking powerful immunosuppressive drugs for other medical conditions. Doctors were alarmed to find a cluster of PCP pneumonia in men who had no reason to have weakened immune systems. The only readily identified trait that these men had in common was that they were all young homosexuals.

Another cluster of 26 men, reported on July 4 of the same year, developed dark, purple splotches on their skin and were found to have Kaposi's sarcoma on their skin biopsies. Kaposi's sarcoma is a cancer caused by a virus that typically causes flat purple tumors, made up of blood vessels, on the skin. Before these cases, this rare form of cancer had mostly been seen in elderly men and was not thought to be very serious. But these men had a different type of Kaposi's sarcoma that was spreading rapidly all over and inside their bodies, and even, in some cases, killing them. Again all were homosexuals, this time between 26 and 51 years old. Tests showed that while parts of the immune system were spared, something was killing these men's helper T cells, a key component of the adaptive immune system, leaving them exposed to infections and tumors not seen in most people. Doctors were left confused and feeling powerless against an unknown medical threat.

Imagine yourself a doctor in New York City in 1981. Until then Kaposi's sarcoma was rare, affecting approximately one in every 2.5 million people. In most cases, the cancer progressed slowly over 10 to 15 years, and Kaposi's sarcoma patients died of something else. The vast majority of doctors would never see a single case. But then you see two cases in one month, both in young men who are on no medications and who have never had major medical problems. Something seems wrong.

You start calling around to other doctors you know, and they've heard of other cases of Kaposi's sarcoma in New York City. Two weeks later you see your two patients again. Their skin cancer is already spreading, and they're complaining that they're losing weight, and that their glands are strangely swollen. What do you do now?

One of the early victims of this new illness was Rick Wellikoff, a 36-year-old homosexual fifth-grade teacher in a disadvantaged Brooklyn neighborhood.

While he worked in Brooklyn, he lived in Greenwich Village with his partner and knew hundreds of people in the local gay community. He had always been healthy until 1979, when he noticed a small, expanding purple pimple on his neck that was diagnosed as Kaposi's sarcoma. His doctor thought this one rare tumor was a freak occurrence until he began inexplicably losing weight and noticed that his lymph nodes were swollen. His friends started to complain, because he would always stay holed up in his apartment and didn't want to come out any more. Soon he had to quit his job because he was always tired, and in 1980 he began to have recurrent bouts of pneumonia, eventually diagnosed as PCP. His Kaposi's sarcoma spread to cover his body and even his internal organs. He deteriorated rapidly, and his friends were shocked when they saw how much weight he had lost over only a few months.

Many medical tests were done, searching in vain for what was destroying his immune system. Tests only revealed that he had a deficiency of T cells, but no explanation could be found. His doctors could not explain to him why he was sick, even as treatment after treatment failed. In December 1980, he fell ill simultaneously with several infections. Realizing that there were no effective medical treatments to help him, he left the hospital two days before Christmas to die at home with his partner in his apartment. His doctors were stunned. He was the fourth American to die of this new mystery disease.

WHERE DID HIV COME FROM?

These patients in the United States were not actually the first cases of HIV. When reports of these men in Los Angeles, San Francisco, and New York began circulating around the globe, doctors remembered other similar, unexplained cases that they had seen. In 1969, a St. Louis teenager known as Robert R. died shortly after coming to the hospital with several infections and difficulty breathing. In the mid-1970s, missionary doctors in Central Africa gave reports of a strange "wasting" disease in which patients lost weight over several years before dying of infections. In 1977, Grethe Rask, a Danish surgeon who worked in Africa, died of PCP. All of these cases confused individual doctors, but the dots were never connected. Nobody suspected that a new disease was to blame until the American cases in 1981.

Research suggests that the most common form of HIV was probably passed from chimpanzees to humans in equatorial Africa between 1902 and 1921. Some primates carry a virus called the simian immunodeficiency virus (SIV). Scientists compared the genetic material from HIV and SIV and have found them remarkably alike. SIV probably jumped from primates into humans in two discrete events. A strain of SIV in the common chimpanzee is closely related to HIV-1, while another strain of SIV in sooty mangabeys is closely related to HIV-2. HIV-1 is the dominant strain of HIV found in the United States and most of the world, while HIV-2 is a generally less virulent, or dangerous, strain found mostly in West Africa. In rare instances, a person can have HIV-1 and HIV-2 at the same time. When people refer to HIV without specifying 1 or 2, they are generally talking about HIV-1, which is far more common in the United States.

Chimpanzees and monkeys used to be hunted and eaten in Africa, and it is thought that at some point a hunter had a cut on his hands that came in contact with chimpanzee blood or that the hunter was bitten and infected with SIV. The infection of a human with SIV probably had to happen many times before the virus transformed into HIV—a human form of this immunodeficiency virus that could then be spread between humans. The fact that SIV was successfully trans-ferred to humans at least twice in the forms of HIV-1 and HIV-2 shows how viruses can actually pass between closely related animals, like humans and primates, and adapt to survive in their new hosts. The first cases of HIV were clustered around Kinshasa (then called Leopoldville) in the Democratic Republic of Congo, which was one of the largest cities in Africa at the time, providing a large enough con-centration of people for the virus to become an epidemic.

HIV probably remained in Central Africa for 20 years before people who were infected traveled outside of that area. During that time the virus most likely mutated many times so that it could pass more easily between people and become more deadly. Because HIV-1 is more infectious and passes more easily between people, it spread out of Africa and around the world. HIV-2 has for the most part remained only in West Africa, although it is also seen in parts of Europe and elsewhere. Eventually HIV-1 moved to Haiti around 1966 before arriving in to the United States approximately four years later. Because people who are infected often don't know they are infected until the late stages of the disease, HIV spread unnoticed in the United States through the 1970s. Asymptomatic carriers spread the virus through "high risk" communities with-out realizing that they were fueling a new epidemic. We will learn more about activities that are considered high risk in chapter 5. By the time the first cases were reported in 1981, thousands of people were already infected.

THE DISEASE SPREADS

Whatever the source, doctors and scientists in the early 1980s were stuck with a new, deadly disease that was quickly killing young, previously healthy people. They started working diligently to find what was destroying the immune systems of their patients. They left no stone unturned as they considered every possible source. Some people thought maybe the patients were taking drugs, and that one batch of drugs had been laced with a toxic substance. Others thought the patients were suffering from a new strain of an old disease, cytomegalovirus. Another possibility considered was that these patients were becoming infected with many diseases at once, overwhelming their immune systems and thereby killing their T cells. Because most of the first patients were homosexuals, the new disease was initially labeled GRID, for Gay-Related Immune Deficiency. A lot of people didn't think that this new disease would infect the heterosexual population, and because of homophobic discrimination they didn't give it much attention.

Soon however, other groups of people started showing signs of AIDS. Injection drug users who shared needles were affected with similar infections. When needles are shared, small amounts of blood can be transferred. Women were getting sick as well, meaning that there was nothing about this new disease that specifically targeted men. On July 9, 1982, the CDC reported a group of 34 Haitians who had recently come to the United States who were sick with rare, serious diseases typically seen in patients with depressed immunity. Half of them had already died, and these men and women denied using injection drugs or being homosexual. It seemed unlikely that a toxic exposure would spread this way to many parts of the country and to other countries affecting groups of people who had no contact with each other. Again, blood from these patients was analyzed and there was a deficiency in the helper T cells of their immune system. This was an infection that was spread not just between men but also between men and women.

Just one week later on July 16, 1982, doctors reported three cases of immune deficiency in hemophiliacs. Hemophiliacs are people who have a rare genetic disorder in which they do not produce enough clotting factors in their blood to stop themselves from bleeding when they are injured. The treatment for a common form of hemophilia for many years was to pool blood from many donors, extract the necessary clotting factor (usually factor VIII), and give the hemophiliac the clotting factor that he or she was missing. However, blood from literally thousands of donors had to be combined to get enough clotting factor. As a result, a hemophiliac would be exposed to blood from hundreds of thousands of anonymous donors during his lifetime. At the time, this pooled blood was screened to remove all known bacteria, fungi, and viruses, but a new virus would not have been detected.

Scientists were now convinced that a virus was somehow attacking people's helper T cells, leaving them vulnerable to infections and causing this new disease. The virus seemed to be spread by bodily fluids, either by sexual contact or blood exposure. And the virus seemed to be spreading quickly. By November 1982, the CDC had gone from reporting 5 isolated cases, to 788 cases in 33 states. In December 1982, the first reports of four infants with immunodeficiency born to infected mothers described a new mechanism of infection: mother-to-child, or "vertical" transmission. People who acquired the virus weren't just getting cancers and pneumonia, but virtually every infection imaginable, in every organ system possible. Doctors were appalled, as countries around the world were beginning to report cases of the newly named disease, AIDS, or acquired immune deficiency syndrome.

SPREAD OF HIV IN AFRICA

Meanwhile, HIV was spreading rapidly, notably in Africa, where the virus originated. In 1985, doctors in Uganda linked what had become known as "slim disease" to reports of AIDS in the United States. Young people in small, rural communities in Africa were literally wasting away, suffering from severe, intractable diarrhea and infections. Slim disease was spreading among sexually active young people and affecting females as frequently as males, rather than targeting homosexual men or injection drug users.

The spread of AIDS accelerated drastically in East Africa, becoming generalized to the entire population at epidemic levels not seen before. Uganda, for example, was severely affected early on. Uganda had a lot of men moving from villages into the city looking for work to support their families. The high proportion of men in the cities, low status of women in Uganda, and large number of prostitutes in some cities led to higher levels of heterosexual transmission. Some retrospective studies showed that in Nairobi, Kenya, the prevalence of HIV among sex workers went from 4 percent in 1981 to over 60 percent in 1985. As you will learn in later chapters, the devastation of the HIV epidemic in Africa would reach terrible proportions.

FINDING THE VIRUS

The race was on to find the virus that was killing T cells and causing AIDS. Scientists in several countries began getting blood samples from patients and isolating T cells. Just a few years earlier, a retrovirus had been discovered that caused T cells to grow uncontrollably as cancer cells. This retrovirus, known as human T-lymphotrophic virus (HTLV), was also spread by sexual contact and blood transfusions and specifically targeted T cells. In some animals, a virus similar to HTLV caused a disease in which the animals lost weight and became prone

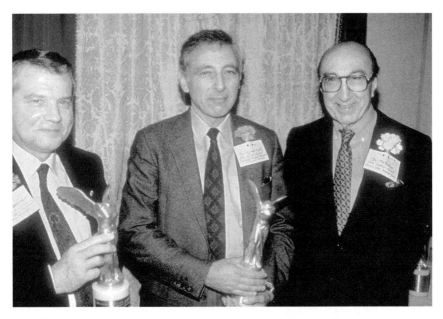

Figure 1.1 (Left to Right) Drs. Luc Montagnier, Robert Gallo, and an uniden-
tified man at an awards ceremony in 1985 for their pioneering work on AIDS
research. (Time & Life Pictures/Getty Images)

to infections. Scientists in the United States and France speculated that a related
virus could be causing AIDS.

One of the first problems faced by the scientists was that by the time patients
clearly had AIDS, many of them didn't have many T cells left. The scientists
learned that most AIDS patients had a period of almost a year when they had
fevers, swollen lymph nodes, and weight loss before they began getting the un-
controlled infections that eventually killed them. So they got samples from the
lymph nodes of patients with swollen nodes and fatigue whom they suspected
would go on to develop full-blown AIDS. They grew the T cells in their labora-
tories and began searching for signs of a new virus.

Their first clue was that the infected T cells contained reverse transcriptase,
the enzyme used by retroviruses to convert their genetic material, called RNA,
into DNA, the form of genetic material in humans. This finding convinced them
that they were searching for a new retrovirus. In May 1983, a French group led
by the scientists Luc Montagnier and Francoise Barre-Sinoussi published that
they had found a new retrovirus from a homosexual man with swollen nodes,
different from HTLV, that they suspected to be the cause of AIDS. They named

the virus lymphadenopathy-associated virus (LAV). At around the same time, an American group led by Peter Gallo found a virus that they thought caused AIDS, using pooled blood from both people with AIDS and a group of men suspected to have an early form of AIDS. The viruses discovered by these two groups were later shown to be exactly the same, but there has been a lot of controversy over which group made the first actual discovery of the new retrovirus. It has generally been agreed that the French group made the initial discovery, paving the way for Montagnier and Barre-Sinoussi to win the 2008 Nobel Prize in Physiology or Medicine. In 1986, a committee decided on the new name human immunodeficiency virus, or HIV.

These landmark findings were confirmed in 1984 as more and more blood samples from people with AIDS were found to contain the new virus. When researchers began testing the blood of patients in Africa with slim disease, they found the same virus recently characterized in France and the United States. The virus was found to specifically attack helper T cells, explaining the dramatic drop in helper T cells seen in patients who were sick with the disease. Many scientists began to optimistically speculate that they would quickly develop a vaccine and AIDS would soon be entirely preventable.

A TEST FOR HIV

While scientists had correctly identified the virus that caused AIDS, they needed to find an effective way to test thousands of people who were at risk of having the disease. People were becoming infected with AIDS after getting blood transfusions, and there needed to be an easy way to test millions of blood samples.

In January 1984, Peter Gallo's lab announced that they had developed a test to detect HIV. The test used an enzyme-linked immunosorbent assay (ELISA) to see if a person had antibodies in their blood that bind to HIV. When a person becomes infected, the immune system works to develop antibodies to the virus. The antibodies recognize parts of the virus and work to clear it from the person's bloodstream. Antibodies are enough to beat many infections, but some HIV viruses remain hidden within cells where B cell antibodies can't see or reach them. Also, HIV is a clever virus that can change the proteins on its own surface—the ones that antibodies target—allowing it to "escape" from antibodies (or the immune system in general). Once a person has been infected by HIV, they have antibodies to the virus for the rest of their lives (even though those antibodies don't control the infection). Because almost nobody clears HIV once they are infected, presence of antibodies almost certainly means that they are infected, with very rare exceptions like HIV vaccine trial participants, or babies who acquire passive transfer of antibodies from their HIV-infected mothers. If those babies are not infected with HIV, the passive antibody is short-lived in their blood. The HIV test was approved by the Food and Drug Administration (FDA) of the U.S. government in 1985 and quickly became available at hospitals around the country.

When an ELISA test is performed, a patient's blood is diluted and passed over a test plate with tiny pieces of HIV, known as antigens. If antibodies are present, they will bind some of these antigens. The plate is then washed clean so that only antibodies bound to antigen remain. An enzyme is applied that both binds the antibodies and becomes fluorescent, so that the antibodies can be seen by a technician. If enough antibody is present, the immunoflourescent signal is strong and the test is considered positive.

The ELISA test is extremely sensitive, meaning that if blood is positive for HIV, it will almost definitely have a positive ELISA test. However, the ELISA test is not considered specific enough, meaning that blood samples negative for HIV will sometimes come out as positive, known as a false positive. This can happen, for example, if a person's blood has a different antibody that "looks like" or "cross-reacts" with the HIV antibody. Even if only one in a hundred tests is a false positive, when you test millions of people for HIV, you will end up telling many people they are HIV positive when they are actually negative.

A second, more expensive test was therefore developed known as the western blot. With the western blot, a sample of the patient's cells are broken up into component proteins and put in a gel where smaller proteins move more quickly than larger proteins. A current is placed across the gel so that the proteins are separated into bands based on size (how much the gel slows them down) and charge (how much they are affected by the current). Once the proteins have all been separated they are transferred onto a membrane. Then the patient's blood is passed over the membrane to see if antibodies in their blood bind pieces of HIV protein, or antigen, from their cells. Again an enzyme is applied that attaches to the antibodies and lights up, allowing a technician to see the result. If specific HIV protein bands are bound by an antibody, the test is considered positive. Western blots are very exact, because several HIV-specific proteins have been separated and bound by the antibodies. For example, one of the HIV surface proteins detected by the western blot is the gp120 protein. As a result, a positive western blot is nearly definitive for a diagnosis of HIV. All patient samples are therefore screened with the cheaper ELISA test first, and the positive ones are then verified with the more expensive, more exact western blot.

The development of these tests changed the face of the AIDS epidemic. Up until this point, only people with serious infections were included in the epidemic.

Suddenly, patients could be tested for HIV infection much earlier in their course of illness, before they developed symptoms of AIDS. Many more people were infected with HIV than had previously been expected. In high-risk populations, the results were shocking. Blood samples from homosexual men taken in 1984 at a sexually transmitted diseases clinic in San Francisco, for example, showed that 140 of 215, or 65 percent, of men were infected. Blood samples from heavy IV drug users in another report showed that 75 of 86, or 87 percent, of recent drug users were infected. Other results showed that 18 out of 25 (72%) hemophiliacs in a home care program were already infected.

When these results were first announced it was speculated that many of these people with HIV would never develop full-blown AIDS. They could even have less dangerous strains of the same disease. For instance, HTLV, the retrovirus related to HIV that causes cancer, only causes symptoms in one in 25 people who have the virus. Eventually, however, it would become clear that almost all of the people with HIV would eventually develop symptoms. The extent of the disease was simply larger than anyone had ever imagined.

One of the major limitations of ELISA and western blot tests is that they are not positive when a person initially becomes infected. Because it takes time for the body to produce the antibodies detected by these two tests, they can initially be falsely negative. In most people it takes two to six weeks to produce antibodies, but in some cases it can take six months or even longer. If a person has been exposed to HIV and wants to be sure they have not contracted the disease, they have to wait up to 6 to 12 months using repeated antibody tests before they can be sure their result is negative.

As a result, other tests for HIV infection have been developed that look for the virus itself, rather than antibodies produced by the body in response to infection. The most common test is one that looks for HIV RNA, to measure a patient's "viral load." The RNA is the genetic material carried in the virus. With this test, RNA is purified out of a patient's blood. This is done by spinning down the blood until all of its components are separated based on their weight. Only the portion with weights similar to RNA is taken and dissolved in water. Then a chemical is added that binds to RNA and makes it sink to the bottom of a glass. Once the RNA has been purified, it is put into a machine and a special test—the polymerase chain reaction (PCR)—is used to amplify only the RNA in the sample that comes from HIV. The PCR can pick out HIV RNA by using what is called a specific HIV primer. If HIV RNA is present, it binds to this primer and amplifies the RNA. This way, even if there is only a very small number of copies of HIV RNA in each milliliter of blood, PCR can amplify these copies until it is more readily detectable. Using this method, technicians can see if the HIV virus itself is in someone's blood. The main limitations of this test are that it is very expensive and time-consuming. It is also more likely to have false positives, for example due to a lab contaminant. This is the downside of a very sensitive PCR test—it can amplify even a contaminant from a splash resulting from a specimen that is placed in a testing well right next to another patient's specimen. The result: someone without HIV may mistakenly be told they are infected. For this reason, doctors usually do not use the HIV viral load alone as a way to diagnose HIV infection. By definition, an HIV antibody test is required.

INITIAL SOCIAL REACTIONS TO HIV

The initial response to AIDS by American authorities was muted at best. The first victims of the new epidemic were groups who were then viewed as on the fringes of society—homosexuals, intravenous drug users, and persons from other countries. While tolerance of homosexuality improved in some cities during the 1970s, it was still not widely acceptable to be openly gay. Intravenous drug users have always been targets of stigma, and many Haitians were seen as outsiders. Scientists initially had difficulty getting funding for their research, even as the AIDS epidemic expanded rapidly. There was relatively little mention in the media during the early 1980s, and many Americans felt that they were immune from this new "gay disease." In the earliest days of the epidemic, the disease didn't even have a name, adding to the fear of the unknown, and labels such as the "gay pneumonia" or "gay-related immune deficiency" (GRID) circulated widely, causing added stigma. As you will see in chapter 8, the history of AIDS is riddled with stories of not only fear and hate, but also courageous bravery and acceptance.

As many politicians preferred to turn a blind eye, it was the infected communities themselves and their supporters who organized teams and worked in unity to start fighting AIDS. In 1981 in New York City, the Gay Men's Health Crisis was formed by people who saw their friends dying and wanted to do more than simply watch helplessly. They raised money, gave a political voice to the terrified men who were getting sick, and started a help hotline to spread information. AIDS activism has been an integral part of fighting the epidemic and giving AIDS victims a voice. Activism has fought apathy and forced governments into action.

SUMMARY

HIV was the result of a "jump" of SIV—a simian immunodeficiency virus—from chimpanzees and sooty mangabeys in Africa to humans, likely in the early 20th century. SIV adapted itself to live in, and be transmitted between, humans at least twice, resulting in HIV-1 and HIV-2. HIV-1 is the more dominant form of HIV infection and is present worldwide, while HIV-2 is typically less aggressive and is generally seen in West Africa or parts of Europe. Initial reports of HIV emerged in 1981 after clusters of previously healthy young people were dying with unusual overwhelming infections or cancers and were found to have a depletion of their helper T cells. The virus was discovered in 1983 and a test for HIV was approved in 1985. This allowed much more rapid identification of persons with HIV infection, even before they developed advanced AIDS. It also allowed protection of the blood supply. Initial social reactions to HIV were characterized by stigma and turning a blind eye, but it soon became clear that HIV was spreading all over the world, as we will see in chapter 4. A strong voice from HIV activists helped to begin fighting the epidemic.

2

What Is HIV?

Kevin J. Selby, MD

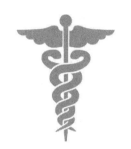

This chapter reviews the basic structure, biology, and human illness caused by the HIV virus. In this chapter we will discuss the following key principles:

- What is HIV?
- What is a virus?
- How does HIV enter the human cell?
- What is the target cell of HIV infection?
- What is the HIV life cycle?
- What is "dormant" HIV?
- How does HIV affect the immune system and cause illness?
- How does HIV escape from immune control?

WHAT IS HIV?

HIV is the abbreviation for Human Immunodeficiency Virus, which infects humans and, if left untreated, causes the Acquired Immune Deficiency Syndrome, AIDS. AIDS is a clinical condition characterized by signs and symptoms that can be diagnosed by a doctor. A person can be defined as having AIDS in one of two ways: either by having complications of a suppressed immune system such as an infection or cancer typically seen in AIDS patients (so called "AIDS-defining illness"), or when blood tests (called the CD4 count) show that the immune system is dangerously weakened reaching a threshold of a CD4 count $\leq$ 200 cells/mm^3. Typically, people are infected with HIV for many years before they develop AIDS. But without treatment, HIV progresses to AIDS, leaving the infected individual with a greatly weakened immune system. In this chapter we will discuss the basic biology of HIV, starting from an explanation of what is a virus, all the way to how HIV suppresses the immune system.

WHAT IS A VIRUS?

A virus is a microscopic infectious agent that depends on host cells to divide and multiply. Each virion (individual virus) is much smaller than a single cell and is composed of genetic material (either DNA or RNA) and a protective protein shell called a capsid. Viruses invade cells and use the host cell machinery to reproduce. Viruses can infect all types of cells, including bacteria, plants, and animals. Viruses were first defined as "filterable agents" because they could escape filtration designed to catch even the smallest bacteria, and then go on to cause infection. Until the 19th century the word *virus* was used to describe anything infectious. Now we know that viruses are just one of many agents that cause infections. Viruses are classified, like bacteria or parasites (other types of infectious organisms), based on their particular biologic characteristics. Viruses are fascinating organisms because they are incredibly efficient in their ability to infect cells, reproduce themselves, and spread infection, but do little else.

Viruses are obligate intracellular parasites. This means that they can only reproduce within other cells. You have probably heard that one way to prevent getting the flu (which is caused by the influenza virus) is to wash your hands frequently. This is because the viruses can exist on inanimate surfaces like doorknobs or subway handles. But they cannot reproduce on these surfaces. To make a copy of itself, a virus must enter a host cell.

When viruses are on their own, they have no way of producing or consuming energy. They are simply made up of genetic material, a protective shell, and proteins that bind the cells they want to invade. They bind target cells and insert their genetic material, using cellular machinery to produce more viruses. In a sense, they put their construction plans into cellular factories of the host that they infect and take command to build what they want to build. They typically carry genetic material for three types of proteins: proteins for copying their own genetic material, proteins that make up the parts of new viruses, and proteins that alter the environment of the cells they invade.

Viruses are different from cellular organisms because they do not divide by binary fission—the process that single-celled organisms use to reproduce—wherein the cell divides into two cells with similar genetic material. More complex organisms like animals reproduce by mixing genetic material and giving birth to offspring. Viruses, as you will see, reproduce by the creation and assembly of different viral components within the cells they infect, that then get packaged up into new viruses that leave the cell ready to infect a new one.

There is debate over whether or not viruses can be considered independent living organisms. While they reproduce and evolve, they have no continuous control over their inner environment and do not consume energy.

Thought Box

What criteria would you suggest to distinguish between living and nonliving organisms? How would you classify: viruses, bacteria, parasites, prions, frozen cells?

Viruses are so tiny that they cannot even be seen with a typical microscope. They are measured in nanometers (nm), or billionths of a meter, a unit of measurement which is far smaller than what you can see with your eyes. A nanometer is one hundred-thousandth of the width of one hair. Viruses are so small that they can generally only be detected by electron microscopes, large research microscopes that "see" by using reflected electrons instead of reflected beams of light as in the more traditional light microscope. Viruses range from just 18nm to 300nm diameter, with HIV landing somewhere in the middle at 80 to 120nm in diameter. As a comparison, most human cells are 7 to 30 *micro*meters, or millionths of a meter, in diameter, which is approximately 300 times bigger in diameter than an HIV virus. A dime is about one *milli*meter thick, or one thousandth of a meter, which is 10,000 times bigger than the diameter of an HIV virus. For the all the problems it causes, HIV is amazingly small!

CASE STUDIES: DIFFERENT TYPES OF VIRUSES

The Common Cold

The effects of viruses on their host range from nearly imperceptible to deadly. Hundreds of viruses infect humans, causing many common and uncommon diseases. The common cold is most often caused by a rhinovirus, a virus that is very well adapted to grow in the moist environment of your nose and mouth.

Rhinoviruses are a type of picornavirus, which tend to be very tough viruses that are easily transmitted by hand-to-hand contact and by contact with nasal secretions. The area of the inside of your nose that is infected by rhinoviruses becomes inflamed and releases fluid, causing you to have a runny nose. You experience cold symptoms until your body manages to fight and overcome the virus. Once that happens, you typically form an antibody to that virus, and the virus is cleared from the body. The immune system is smart and keeps a "track record" of essentially all the infections it has seen before, encoded in the immune cells. In this way the body "remembers" if you encounter that virus again and is able to rapidly mount a strong response against that virus. But there are over 100 types of rhinovirus, which is part of the reason why it is almost impossible to become immune to the common cold. This means we can get a cold season after season even though we've had one before.

The Chicken Pox (Varicella) Virus

Another virus, the varicella-zoster virus (VZV), is a type of herpes virus that causes both chicken pox (also called varicella) and, when it recurs, shingles (also called zoster), typically occurring later in life. Chicken pox (or initial VZV infection) is generally transmitted from one person to another through the air or by contact with the infectious rash. When inhaled by someone who is not immune to chicken pox (by either having had the illness before or by having received a vaccine against chicken pox), the virus enters the respiratory tract and then infects and divides in the cells of the lungs. People who have chicken pox are infectious to others a few days before the rash even appears through this mechanism. Once the rash appears, contact with the rash can also spread the disease. VZV is also contagious when it shows up as zoster, the reactivation form of this virus. Zoster causes a classic rash with painful red blisters. The skin lesions of zoster are infectious and shouldn't be touched.

VZV is extremely infectious and will spread to up to 90 percent of household contacts who have never been infected or had the vaccine. The course of primary infection is as follows: after three or four days it spreads into the blood and infects different organs like the liver and spleen. Soon after, the virus causes a fever, a general feeling of fatigue, and a spotty rash. The rash is characterized by many tiny blisters, classically described by doctors as having the appearance of a "dewdrop on a rose petal." A small vesicle, or bubble of fluid, is surrounded by red inflammation of the skin. These spots, as anyone who has ever had chicken pox can tell you, are incredibly itchy and appear in batches over three to five days. They are caused by localized infection and killing of skin cells. A person with a chicken pox rash is considered infectious until the rash is crusted over.

The immune system develops immunity to VZV but, in comparison to the common cold, almost never manages to clear it completely from the body. Instead, the virus "hides" in a dormant state in nerve cells near the spinal cord called dorsal root ganglia. Viruses like VZV are able to remain latent in your body. The dormant state, as its name implies, means that the virus is resting or sleeping quietly. Because it is not actively replicating or causing overt illness, the person may have no symptoms at all, but the virus is still present in the nerve cells and can reactivate later in time.

As we get older, immunity to VZV can slowly wane. Sometimes the immune system can get weaker for a number of other reasons beyond aging. These include certain medications such as steroids, immunosuppressive drugs, or chemotherapeutic agents; and certain conditions like diabetes, organ or bone marrow transplantation, cancer, or HIV infection, among others. Some people even think that stress alone can weaken the immune system enough to allow VZV reactivation. Under such circumstances, VZV can reemerge and cause a very painful rash known as shingles or zoster. The virus travels from the nerve cell nucleus (where it was previously dormant) down to the nerve endings near the surface of the skin, classically producing a rash in the specific area of skin affected by those nerves. The exact location and distribution of the rash therefore depends on which dorsal root ganglion the virus initially resides in. Because each part of the skin is innervated by a particular set of nerves, doctors can usually tell where the virus is hiding out by tracing back the site of the rash to the nerves that supply that part of the skin. A common place to see zoster is on the trunk, usually along the ribs on one side of the body. Another common place is on the face, often involving one side of the forehead and the tip of the nose. Shingles most commonly appears only on one side of the body.

Ebola Virus

Some other viruses are more rare but can cause very extreme, deadly symptoms. The Ebola virus is a type of filovirus that can cause a severe, often fatal illness called hemorrhagic fever. It gets this name because it creates extreme fragility of blood vessels, resulting in potentially fatal bleeding episodes. The virus is transmitted to humans from fruit bats in Central Africa and can then spread from human to human through contact with infected blood or bodily fluids. The virus initially causes very common symptoms like fevers and headaches. However, it replicates extremely quickly and causes breakdown in the function of organs like the kidneys, liver, and spleen. Soon it invades the walls of blood vessels and causes massive internal bleeding. Very scary indeed! One outbreak in the Democratic Republic of Congo had an almost 90 percent mortality (death) rate within two weeks. Luckily the virus is rare and remote and is only transmitted by infected biologic material. Because it quickly causes symptoms, it is easier to identify before it goes on to infect many other people, compared to a virus that is harder to "see" because it doesn't make its host sick right away.

As you can see, different viruses have evolved different ways of infecting and affecting humans. Some are very hardy and common but relatively mild; others are very deadly but relatively rare. Some are short lived: they cause illness and then disappear once the immune system gains control of the infection. Others persist, remaining dormant in our bodies even years after the initial infection. Which of these characteristics, or other characteristics, do you think describe HIV?

THE STRUCTURE OF HIV

The Human Immunodeficiency Virus, HIV, is the most common member of its family of viruses—"retroviruses." Retroviruses are roughly spherical in shape, with an envelope (or lipid membrane) around their "capsid," or protective protein shell (see Figure 2.1). The envelope is composed of fats and proteins. An envelope makes it easier for HIV to enter human cells, and to avoid immune system detection. However, having an envelope also makes HIV more sensitive to breakdown by detergents, heat, or dry conditions. As a result, HIV is actually quite delicate and does not survive well outside of humans. Unlike influenza viruses, it cannot survive very long on its own in the environment, for example on your hands, clothes, or in the air.

In nearly all forms of life, genetic material is encoded as either DNA (deoxyribonucleic acid) or RNA (ribonucleic acid). The blueprints needed to make a new HIV virus are encoded in RNA. The envelope and capsid surround the HIV RNA. Both RNA and DNA are long chains of four different kinds of bases in a precise order to encode for the proteins that make up our cells. Each three bases in a row encode a specific amino acid, which are linked together as the building blocks of proteins. DNA is the more stable, permanent form of genetic material found in each one of our cells. Human DNA is organized in 46 chromosomes and is kept in the cell nucleus. It is generally only copied very carefully when cells are dividing. Also, DNA is double stranded, meaning that each strand is bound to a complementary copy of itself to add stability and a spare copy of the genetic

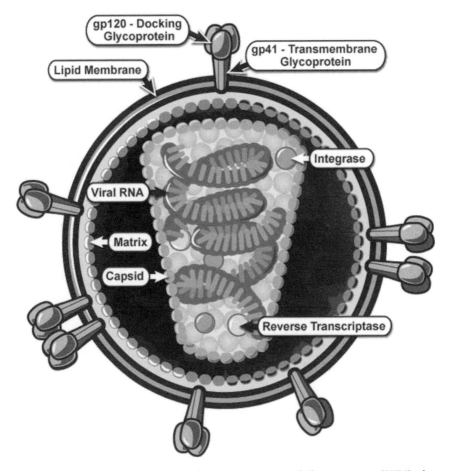

Figure 2.1 Schematic drawing of the human immunodeficiency virus (HIV), the virus that causes AIDS. (National Institute of Allergy and Infectious Diseases)

material. However, as we shall see, human DNA has to be transcribed into RNA before a protein can be made.

Role of DNA and RNA in Reproduction

During mitosis or cell division, DNA makes copies of itself so that each new cell has exactly the same component of DNA, arranged in 46 chromosomes. The only exception is in human gametes—eggs in females and sperm in males. These cells are formed by a process called meiosis, which results in cells that have only half the usual complement of DNA, arranged in 23 chromosomes. When an egg and a sperm unite, the resulting cell has the full complement of 46 chromosomes and can go on to divide and create new cells.

In addition to its central role in cell division, DNA is the blueprint that dictates the synthesis of many different proteins. To make new proteins, DNA is transcribed into single-stranded RNA, which is then translated into a protein. RNA is the form of genetic information generally used temporarily to provide the template for new proteins. Messenger RNA is the bridge between DNA and new proteins. Transfer RNA is the "decoder" that "reads" messenger RNA three bases at a time and links specific amino acids (the building blocks of proteins) to the growing protein chain coded for by that messenger RNA.

All retroviruses contain RNA as their genetic code, but some other viruses (hepatitis B virus, for example), contain DNA. Because DNA and RNA are made up of bases in a precise sequence, we refer to the length of RNA or DNA in numbers of bases in the chain. The HIV genome is about 9,000 base pairs long. By comparison, the human genome is three billion base pairs long. HIV has just 9 genes, compared to around 20,000 to 25,000 genes found in a human. Suffice to say that making a human being is a little more complicated than making a virus.

The core of the HIV virus also contains two enzymes. Enzymes are specially designed proteins that speed up and facilitate the chemical reactions and interactions that occur in cells. All of the processes in cells, from the generation of energy to division, depend on enzymes. Usually viruses "hijack" enzymes from the cells they infect, but HIV comes packaged with two of its own enzymes that aren't usually present in human cells. The enzymes are reverse transcriptase (RT) and integrase. You will learn about their function later in the book.

On the outer surface of the HIV virus are the glycoproteins that bind to target cells. Glycoproteins are proteins that also contain sugar chains. They are named based on their size. The two most important glycoproteins on the surface of HIV are gp41 and gp120. These form lollipop-like spikes on the surface of the virus and bind to receptors on the surface of target cells (see Figure 2.1).

INFECTION WITH HIV

HIV infection begins with entry of the virus into human target cells, marking successful HIV transmission. HIV transmission can happen through several different routes, but it most frequently happens during sexual intercourse or direct inoculation of virus into the blood (by intravenous drug use, for example). The details of HIV transmission will be covered in chapter 5, but we will talk about the basics here. HIV can be transmitted sexually, through infected blood products or bodily fluids, or from a mother to her baby. Because HIV is very delicate, it must rapidly come into contact with its target cells for transmission to occur.

HIV Receptors

HIV targets several different immune cells, including T lymphocytes, monocyte/macrophage cells, and dendritic cells. Only certain cells have the right receptors for HIV to bind. HIV needs two receptors: CD4 and either CCR5 or CXCR4. CD4 is a coreceptor used to activate immune cells, while CCR5 and CXCR4 are chemokine coreceptors that normally bind to signals between immune cells but can also serve as HIV receptors. CCR5 is usually most important during initial infection. Later in the course of disease CXCR4 can become an important coreceptor.

When HIV bumps into an immune cell, gp120—a viral envelope glycoprotein—binds to the CD4 receptor on the human cell and anchors the virus to the cell (see Figure 2.2). The binding of gp120 causes this glycoprotein to change shape, which then allows it to bind CCR5 on the host cell at the same time, and expose the next HIV molecule, gp41, which is hidden underneath. The newly exposed gp41 binds to the surface of the cell and draws together the viral envelope and the cell membrane, allowing them to fuse together. Very precise pictures of gp41 have shown that it actually pushes through the cell membrane of the target cell and coils upon itself to bring the virus and the cell together. Once the membranes have fused, the viral capsid is in. It has broken through the first level of defense.

One of the ways that scientists recognized the importance of CCR5 in HIV transmission was the discovery of the so called "CCR5 delta 32 mutation," found in about one percent of Caucasians. Persons who have this mutation in the CCR5 receptor were found to be more resistant to HIV infection. There were reports of rare individuals who had repeated sexual exposure to a certain strain of HIV but did not become infected. Genetic analysis showed that they had a 32-base-pair section missing from both copies of their CCR5 gene, making them homozygous for this mutation. Individuals with only one delta-32 gene, so-called heterozygous for that trait, appear to also have a somewhat lower likelihood of infection and may show slower disease progression if they are infected. Up to 20 percent of people in some European countries are heterozygous for the CCR5 delta-32 mutation. Blood testing from Africa and Asia has shown that delta-32 mutations are either extremely rare or absent in those populations.

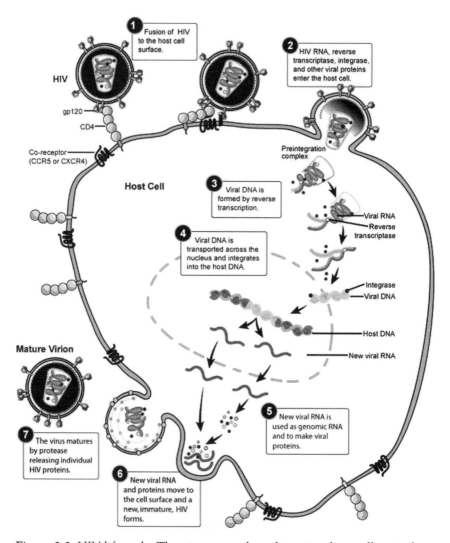

Figure 2.2 HIV life cycle. The virus can only replicate in a host cell, using host machinery. (National Institute of Allergy and Infectious Diseases)

Some scientists speculate that not having CCR5 mutations in those areas of the world may have contributed to more widespread HIV epidemics. Unfortunately, people with C delta-32 mutations can still become infected with some less common strains of HIV, for example those that use the CXCR4 receptor right at the onset of infection.

VIRAL LIFE CYCLE 1: HACKING INTO THE CELL

Once the viral capsid is inside its target cell, it begins to move towards the cell nucleus. At this point one of the enzymes inside the viral capsid, reverse transcriptase, begins to work. Reverse transcriptase copies the HIV RNA into DNA. It is called reverse transcriptase because usually DNA is copied into RNA, but HIV works in reverse. Humans don't have reverse transcriptase in any of their cells, because our genomic material is encoded in DNA in each cell nucleus, and we don't have any need to change RNA into DNA. After the HIV RNA has been copied into DNA, the reverse transcriptase breaks down the old RNA and makes a complementary strand for the new DNA so that it is double stranded. The DNA version of the HIV RNA genome is also called cDNA or copy DNA.

HIV Reverse Transcriptase: Accident Prone

One characteristic of HIV reverse transcriptase is that it makes a lot of mistakes. HIV reverse transcriptase makes about one error per 2,000 to 4,000 base pairs, which adds up to roughly two to five mistakes every time the 9,000-base-pair genome is copied. In comparison, when human DNA is copied to allow for cell division, there is less than one mistake per million base pairs. Considering the fact that up to 10 billion copies of HIV are made every day in an HIV-infected person, two to five mistakes per copy adds up quickly. Mistakes in the DNA eventually cause changes in the proteins encoded by that DNA sequence. These mistakes, called mutations, are then passed along in the newly made viruses as they replicate. Most of these mutations are in locations that have no effect on the function of the virus. Some of the mutations actually create viruses that are nonfunctional and cannot go on to infect other cells, meaning that the viral replication is less efficient than it could be. But every once in a while, one of these mutations makes a new virus that is resistant to drugs or can evade the human immune system by altering the viral protein product that the immune system targets. By having a high error rate, HIV can mutate and evolve quickly, allowing it to change the face that it shows the immune system.

HIV cDNA

Once the DNA copy of the HIV genome has been made, it passes through pores, or holes, to get into the nucleus. Here the enzyme integrase inserts the HIV DNA into the cell's DNA (see Figure 2.2). Integrase is the other enzyme carried by the virus in its capsid. Once the DNA has been added, it is indistinguishable from the rest of the cell's DNA. This DNA carries the code for all of the proteins and RNA that make up the HIV virus. Now when the infected cell is activated, it will produce not only its own proteins, but HIV proteins as well. The virus has broken into the cell's control room and slipped its plans into the cell's blueprints; by doing so it turns the cell into a factory for virus parts that can then be assembled into new viruses.

VIRAL LIFE CYCLE 2: VIRAL PRODUCTION

Active vs. Dormant States of HIV

Once the viral genetic material has become part of the cell's DNA, two things can happen. If the cell is inactive, the HIV infection becomes a latent infection. In this state, the viral DNA is stably integrated and the cell is indistinguishable from a noninfected cell to the immune surveillance system (which is continuously probing for "foreigners" that endanger the body). The integrated virus is also invisible to HIV medications, which predominantly target replicating viruses, and is therefore unaffected by them. This type of latent infection makes it nearly impossible to "cure" someone of HIV. Even just one remaining latent virus is able to emerge from its dormant state, make copies of itself, and rekindle infection. The latent or dormant state is established as early as 72 hours after infection.

Active Replication

If the cell is active, it will be actively transcribing DNA into RNA and producing its own proteins. During the earliest phases of HIV infection, the body's immune system is seeing HIV for the first time and becomes very active. As a result, many of the immune cells targeted by HIV are active. If the virus enters one of these activated immune cells, it will produce enormous amounts of viral proteins. HIV is a complex virus, in that its genetic material not only contains coding for the final structure of the virus, but also extra proteins that act as regulatory proteins. These regulatory proteins encourage the cell to produce more viral proteins, help with the processing of the new proteins, and promote maturation of the new viruses as they are assembled.

Viral proteins begin to accumulate in the cytoplasm of the infected cell. The proteins go out toward the surface of the cell and get assembled into new viruses. Some of the proteins are transported so that they extend through the cell membrane, serving as "flags" to the immune system that that cell is infected with

HIV. Remember that latently infected cells are not replicating, do not form viral proteins, and therefore are "unmarked," leaving the immune system blind to the HIV infection. In contrast, activated cells give the immune system an opportunity to recognize the HIV invader and activate an immune response to try to contain the virus.

In a replicating cell, the capsid assembles from structural proteins into a complex shell that encircles newly formed HIV RNA. Some of the enzymes that will form part of the new virus, like newly formed reverse transcriptase, are initially created with several proteins attached together. An enzyme called protease cuts these new proteins into their right size and shape. Part of the cell membrane begins budding off from the rest of the cell membrane, surrounding a newly assembled capsid. A newly formed HIV virus then breaks off from the surface of the cell and is free to infect other cells and continue the viral life cycle (see Figure 2.2). This process doesn't necessarily kill the cell, but oftentimes so much of the cell's resources become devoted to producing virus that it dies. The cell may also die because the immune system, recognizing the invader "flags" on its surface, targets it for destruction. Because HIV targets immune cells for infection, each cell death leaves an infected individual slightly more susceptible to other infections.

SUMMARY

HIV is a clever virus that attacks the human immune system. It uses the host cell machinery to make copies of itself. The newly made viruses bud from the infected cell and go on to invade other cells. HIV comes packaged with its own "reverse transcriptase"—an enzyme that helps it to replicate itself. The reverse transcriptase makes a lot of mistakes, resulting in the opportunity for changes in the HIV genome that may allow it to evade the immune system or escape from drugs that target the virus. HIV can replicate in an active cell or stay dormant in an inactivated cell, integrated into the human host cell DNA. When it is dormant, it is not replicating, but it is also "invisible" to the immune system and to the drugs that target replicating HIV.

3

An Introduction to the Human Immune System

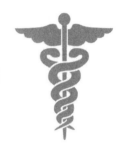

Kevin J. Selby, MD

This chapter reviews the basics of the immune system—its key components and how it works. In this chapter we will explore the following questions:

- How is the immune system structured?
- What is innate versus adaptive immunity?
- Which cells are the key players in the immune system? What roles do they play?
- How does the immune system respond to HIV infection?
- How does HIV weaken the immune system?
- What are the clinical laboratory markers of HIV infection (including CD4 count and viral load)?
- What is the difference between HIV and AIDS?
- What are "opportunistic infections"?

As we mentioned before, HIV only infects certain cells, such as T lymphocytes, monocyte/macrophage cells, and dendritic cells. These cells are part of the body's intricate immune system, which helps prevent infections and some cancers. Our immune systems have evolved over millions of years to keep up with the microbes that are continuously creating new ways of infecting us. An intact immune system is critical, as our physical environment is filled with microbes trying to get into the warm, protected environment inside our body.

Thought Box

Human beings live in balance with microbes. The immune system fights off dangerous microbial invaders, but some microbes live in a healthy balance with humans. Can you think of examples of bacteria that are normally found in humans? Where do they live? How do they survive? What role do they play in their human host?

AIDS, when untreated, depresses the immune system and leaves its human hosts vulnerable to dozens of usually harmless diseases. The immunosuppression caused by untreated AIDS highlights the importance of a healthy immune system. Any person's immune system has to find a delicate balance between attacking foreign invaders and not harming its own self. A hyperactive immune system can cause autoimmune diseases, allergic reactions, or medical problems from a chronic "inflammatory state."

THE TWO ARMS OF THE IMMUNE SYSTEM: INNATE VS. ADAPTIVE IMMUNITY

Our defense against infections has two parts: innate immunity and adaptive immunity. Innate immunity, also called intrinsic or native immunity, is a powerful early defense mechanism that attacks microbes and clears debris as soon as they are seen by cells in the innate system. All multicellular organisms have intrinsic mechanisms for preventing infections. The most basic part of our innate immune system is our skin and the lining of our lungs and intestines, which come into contact with microbes every day from direct contact, inhalation, or swallowing, for example. These tissues therefore have specialized cells to recognize and trap foreign particles. In addition to physical barriers like the hair and mucus in our noses, the respiratory system has specialized immune cells to recognize and fight infections. There are many cell types in the innate immune system, including phagocytes, dendritic cells, and natural killer cells. Phagocytes attack by engulfing and eating invaders or debris like human Pac-mans! In fact, the name *phagocyte* is derived from the Greek work *phagos*—which means "eat."

The adaptive immune system develops over time, responding to the invaders that it sees in the body. It is an intricate system that requires the coordination of

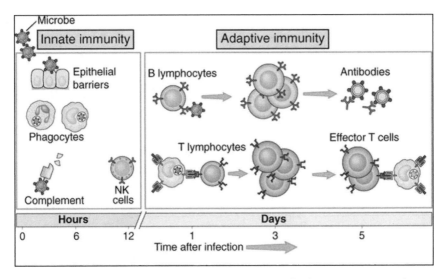

Figure 3.1 Schematic drawing of different types of cells that participate in the innate or adaptive arms of the immune system. (Adapted from Abbas and Lichtman: *Basic Immunology*, 3rd edition.)

many different types of soldiers in the immune system but is often much more specific to the enemy that it is targeting than the more "blunt" effect of the innate immune system. Another difference is that the effects of the innate immune system are generally short-lived, while those of adaptive immunity have a much longer impact, owing to special cells called memory cells, which we'll learn about soon.

Innate Immune System

The innate immune system recognizes structures that are shared by some microbes but are not present on host cells. For example, many bacteria produce a substance in their cell membranes called lipopolysaccharide, but mammals do not. Sometimes the immune system encounters bacteria outside cells, recognizes them as foreigners, and can activate part of the innate immune system called "complement," which facilitates destruction of the bacteria. If the bacteria have invaded a cell, parts of the bacteria will be shuttled up to the cell surface and displayed as flags to help the immune system know that that particular cell has been infected. Phagocytes can recognize lipopolysaccharide or other specific bacterial parts displayed on the infected cell, and are therefore triggered to eat that cell. They also recognize more general debris and engulf the foreign material directly. The phagocyte literally ingests bacteria or infected cells and degrades them into little pieces.

Adaptive Immune System

While the innate immune system supplies an immediate, blunt response, adaptive immunity develops more slowly and supplies a later, more effective, and longer-lasting defense against infections. There are two types of adaptive immunity: humoral immunity and cell-mediated immunity. Humoral immunity uses antibodies produced by B cells, while cell-mediated immunity depends largely on T cells (see Figure 3.2).

Phagocytes form an important link with the adaptive immune system. Once they have degraded a foreign body, they present the pieces to cells of the adaptive

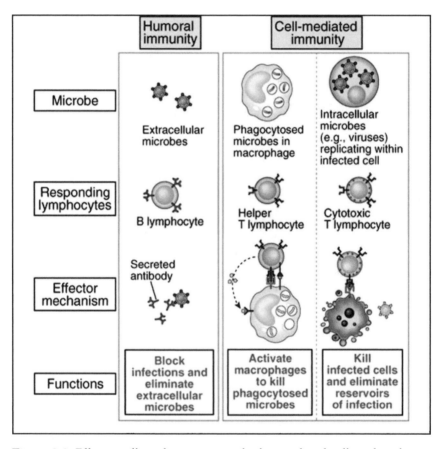

Figure 3.2 Effector cells and activities in the humoral and cell-mediated arms of the adaptive immune system. (Adapted from Abbas and Lichtman: *Basic Immunology*, 3rd edition.)

immune system for analysis. These small pieces, called antigens, are what trigger a wider immune response. The phagocytes go out and ingest particles they recognize as foreign and present their findings to the adaptive immune system. When they are playing this role, we call them antigen-presenting cells (APCs). The APCs can bring their information to "surveillance centers" like lymph nodes. The cells of the adaptive immune system process the information in a way that allows the body to mount a large and orchestrated immune response with many soldier cells of the adaptive immune system, if the body encounters that antigen again. Here's how they do it.

B and T Cells

Both B and T cells are lymphocytes and use a similar principle to fight diseases. These lymphocytes circulate in the body, routinely moving through surveillance lymph nodes to see if antigen-presenting cells have found a microbe with an antigen that fits their binding site. If a lymphocyte encounters such an antigen, it then divides into thousands of mature lymphocytes that can attack one specific microbe. In this way lymphocytes are able to adapt to specifically attack invading microbes.

One of the distinguishing features of the adaptive immune system is that it has memory cells. Once lymphocytes for a specific infection have successfully cleared that microbe from the body, most of the specific lymphocytes die off. But some of them stick around as memory lymphocytes, ready if a similar microbe ever reappears. If a similar microbe causes an infection again, the adaptive immune system will have a faster, stronger response the second time, often stopping an infection before it becomes widespread enough to cause symptoms. The first time your adaptive immune system is exposed to a new microbe, it can take several weeks to mount a complete immune response. The next time it is exposed to the same microbe, it will respond within days or even faster, and repeated exposures often speed up and intensify the immune response. Vaccines work by "showing" the immune system particles that resemble infections, prompting it to create memory lymphocytes against that infection, so that a vaccinated individual can stop an infection like measles before it even causes symptoms. Memory cells can rapidly trigger the production and release of many antibodies directed specifically at the particular infection the "remember."

Autoimmune Disease

Great care is taken by your adaptive immune system to ensure that it doesn't mistakenly identify molecules from your own body as foreign and mount a misguided immune response. When lymphocytes are being developed they are exposed to particles from all around your body. If the lymphocytes bind too tightly to the "self" antigen, it does not fully develop. As well, when a lymphocyte encounters a foreign particle, there have to be surrounding signs of inflammation in order to begin an immune response. This is another layer of protection from attacking self, since our own antigens and tissues are usually not surrounded by inflammation unless there is a harmful infection or injury. However, sometimes mistakes happen, and the immune system attacks self-antigens, resulting in autoimmune diseases such as type I diabetes and rheumatoid arthritis. Can you think of other autoimmune diseases and imagine what kind of self-antigen is being attacked?

Antibodies

As mentioned above, B cells are in charge of humoral immunity. Their key weapon is antibodies. Antibodies are Y-shaped molecules with a special region at the end of each arm that can bind foreign proteins, fats, and sugars. B cells have antibodies on their surface with a specific binding site. If the B cell binds with its antigen, it becomes activated. The B cell then divides rapidly and begins producing many more free-floating antibodies that bind to invading microbes, impairing their function and targeting them for destruction. In most cases B cells actually require stimulation by T cells to have full activation.

Cell-Mediated Immunity

T cells are in charge of the cell-mediated immunity, which plays a role against microbes that are inside of your cells, either because they have infected that cell, or because that cell ingested the microbe to break it down. There are two main types of T cells: CD4 T cells, also known as helper T cells, and CD8 T cells, known as cytotoxic T cells. They are named for the CD4 and CD8 receptors on their surfaces. You may remember that CD4 T cells are the ones targeted most often by HIV. Cell-mediated immunity has another important role: it provides a special surveillance to help in prevent the development of some cancers. When T cells are in this role, they are called "tumor surveillance" cells.

CD4 Helper Cells

CD4 cells are called helper T cells because they "help" activate other parts of the immune system. They are not phagocytic (i.e., they do not "eat" other cells or microbes) or cytolytic (i.e., they do not destroy or break down other cells), but instead they coordinate the rest of the immune system to respond to an infection. When CD4 cells become activated, they secrete cytokines, which are tiny molecules that signal to the rest of the immune system that an infection or inflammation is occurring. Cytokines recruit more blood flow and immune cells to the area of infection. When you see red inflammation around a cut that becomes infected, that is cytokines at work, increasing blood flow to the area so that immune cells can aid in the healing process. CD4 cells can activate B cells to make antibodies. CD4 cells also activate the phagocytic cells of the innate immune system to become more active, ingest more microbes, and lyse—or break up—the microbes. Finally, CD4 cells also activate CD8 cells, which have cytolytic (or cell killing) activity. CD4 cells are activated by the antigen-presenting cells of the innate immune system when these cells recognize a foreign particle and present them to a CD4 cell.

Cytotoxic T Cells

CD8 cells are called cytotoxic or cytolytic T cells because they can kill other cells. Once a CD8 cell has been activated to look for a certain antigen, any cell that is producing or displaying that antigen will be killed. For instance, if a CD8 cell were activated to recognize the gp120 protein on the surface of HIV, any cell that is infected and actively making HIV viruses will display small pieces of gp120, an HIV antigen, on its cell surface. A CD8 cell recognizes the antigen and binds tightly to the infected cells. It then releases toxic chemicals that result in death of the infected cell.

EFFECT OF HIV ON THE IMMUNE SYSTEM

When someone with a normal immune system at baseline initially becomes infected with HIV, the immune system quickly rises to the challenge of detecting and responding to this new invader. The innate immune system will ingest many HIV particles and begin activating the adaptive immune system. The first weeks of infection are a race between the virus and the immune system, as the immune system activates NK cells and phagocytes, works to produce B and T cells in order to have antibodies that coat free virus, CD4 helper T cells to activate other components of the immune response, and CD8 cells to kill infected cells. A newly infected patient will experience fevers, diffuse pains, and fatigue as their immune system uses large amounts of the body's resources to combat the new infection. These symptoms are often caused by the cytokines that are released during all of this massive immune activation.

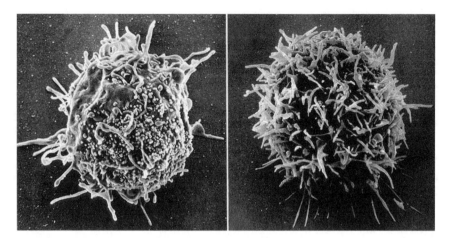

Figure 3.3 The image on the right is a normal T cell, which defends the immune system from infection. The image on the left is an HIV-infected T cell. (National Library of Medicine)

In many other infections, the immune system is well adapted and works fast enough to beat the infection. But HIV is different. First, HIV targets the CD4 cells that lead the immune response, so that even relatively early in an infection, the immune system is weakened by injury to one of its key components. Second, HIV incorporates its genetic information into the DNA of infected cells and can cause latent infection, as we described earlier. Latent infections are not detected by the immune system and can go unnoticed. Eventually, these latent cells begin to produce viral particles, and the infection continues at low levels initially, building to higher and more destructive levels later in the course of infection. Finally, HIV has the ability to change its appearance by creating changes in its envelope proteins as a result of its error prone reverse transcriptase. This means that it can more readily escape from the immune system, because it is continuously looking for a virus that keeps changing its appearance.

HIV's Effect on CD4 Cells

HIV binds to CD4 to enter cells, so its primary target is helper T cells. Over time, there is a progressive loss of CD4 cells. In some parts of the body, like the gut, for example, the initial depletion of CD4 cells can be profound and difficult to recover. A normal person has about 500–1,500 CD4 cells per microliter (μL) of blood, although this number is somewhat variable. Eventually, if HIV is not treated, the number of CD4 cells will dwindle down to 200 cells per μL, usually over the course of several years. If untreated, HIV will cause the loss of approximately 100 CD4 cells per year on average (some people have a faster or slower rate of decline, depending on how well their bodies can control HIV). As a result, an infected individual becomes progressively prone to more and more infections. The cell-mediated immunity of CD4 cells primarily prevents some bacterial and viral infections, mycobacterial infections (like tuberculosis), and cancer. HIV-infected patients get sick from infections that would not usually cause harm in someone with normal levels of CD4 cells, or that would cause less pronounced disease in individuals with healthy immune systems; we call these infections opportunistic infections.

Opportunistic Infections

Opportunistic infections can result from microbes that are very common in our environment, but that are usually dealt with easily by a healthy immune system. Pneumocystis pneumonia (PCP) is a good example. It is caused by *Pneumocystis jirovecii*, an intracellular fungus that is ubiquitous in our environment. Any one of us may encounter PCP, but HIV patients with very low CD4 cells become unable to fight off PCP, and it can cause a serious lung infection. You will learn more about opportunistic infections in chapter 6.

FROM HIV TO AIDS

AIDS, as you may remember from an earlier chapter, is a syndrome. Syndromes are associated signs (which the doctor can see), symptoms (which the patient can feel), and certain laboratory test results that can occur in typical patterns. An infection simply means that you have a particular microbe in your body, but it may or may not be producing symptoms, signs, or abnormal lab results at any given time. Latent HIV and early tuberculosis are examples of infections that may not produce symptoms at first.

Having AIDS means that the immune system is suppressed to the extent that meets certain criteria set by a panel of experts. If someone is infected with HIV, their doctor will decide if they meet the definition of AIDS. The criteria for defining AIDS includes a CD4 count less than 200 or the presence of a so-called AIDS-defining illness. You will learn more about these in a later chapter. If an HIV infection is left untreated, it weakens a patient's immune system to the point that he or she will have signs and symptoms that we call AIDS. AIDS is very dangerous because it is characterized by a severely damaged immune system and many infections that can be fatal.

One of the ways to tell if someone is progressing toward having AIDS is to test the level of damage done by HIV to that person's immune system. The easiest way to do that is to measure how many CD4 cells they have in their blood. This measurement is referred to as a CD4 count and is a key clinical laboratory marker of HIV disease. It tells doctors about the relative strength of the immune system. Someone with a high CD4 count (more than 200), and no opportunistic infections or other AIDS-defining illnesses (like certain cancers or other complications) is defined as having HIV disease. When the CD4 count falls below 200, or the course of illness progresses to include certain infections or complications, the disease is defined as AIDS. When someone's CD4 count is below 350 (some experts even say 500), they become more susceptible to many infections, as the immune system is already weakened.

The other key clinical laboratory marker of HIV disease and its progression is a test called the viral load. This test measures the amount of HIV copies in the blood. The viral load is higher when the virus is replicating more actively. It is also a marker for transmission risk, since higher viral loads are also associated with a greater degree of infectivity. The goal of treatment is to get the viral load to undetectable levels, but it may rise when medications are no longer effective, due to the emergence of viral resistance, for example. We will explore the details of treatment and resistance in chapter 7.

SUMMARY

The immune system is a complex structure that is designed to protect us against microscopic invaders. It has two main arms: innate and adaptive immunity. The immune system has several "soldiers," including natural killer cells, phagocytes, T cells, and B cells. T cells include both CD4 and CD8 cells. HIV infects CD4 cells and impairs their function. HIV infection progresses to AIDS when the CD4 count falls below 200 cells/μL or when the immune system is substantially weakened and the patient suffers from typical AIDS-defining illnesses.

4

HIV around the World (Global Epidemiology)

Sigall K. Bell, MD

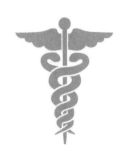

This chapter describes estimates of HIV prevalence around the world, incidence of new infections, and basic epidemiologic principles describing the dynamics of disease spread. We will explore the following questions:

- What part of the world has the greatest burden of HIV infection?
- What is the estimate of the total number of adults and children living with HIV in the United States, and different countries around the world?
- What is an epidemic?
- When does a disease become an epidemic?
- What can we learn from different models of infection, for example comparing HIV to measles?
- What is the basic reproductive rate of infection?
- What factors determine whether a disease will spread, remain contained, or be eradicated?
- How do we define common epidemiologic terms like *prevalence* and *incidence*?

While HIV is present worldwide, the greatest burden of disease is by far concentrated in sub-Saharan Africa. Of an estimated 34 million cases of HIV globally in 2008, 22–23 million were in sub-Saharan Africa. In contrast, it is estimated that approximately 1.4 million people are currently living with HIV in North America. Of the total global infections, 2 million are in children under the age of 15. Of the 3 million new global infections in 2008, 2 million occurred in sub-Saharan Africa. Of the roughly 2 million deaths from HIV/AIDS globally in 2008, 1.4 occurred in sub-Saharan Africa.

These figures suggest that there were an average of 7,400 new HIV infections across the world each day in 2008 (including 1,200 children under the age of 15 infected each day). Ninety-seven percent of these occurred in low and middle-income countries. Despite the decrease in AIDS cases owing to the use of HIV treatment, and the dramatic decline in HIV/AIDS deaths, the number of new infections has held steady at about 50,000 cases/year in the United States. The lack of decline suggests a failure in primary prevention. Effective delivery of educational messages and reduction in high-risk behavior that increases the chances of being infected with HIV requires increased attention.

There is concern that the rate of high-risk behavior has not only failed to decrease, it has actually increased. This concern is a result of increased reported cases of gonorrhea and syphilis in some states, especially among populations of men who have sex with men. Given the shared mode of transmission (unprotected sexual intercourse) and the increased risk of HIV transmission in the presence of genital ulcer disease, these trends are particularly concerning. We will further discuss issues related to transmission in chapter 5.

WHAT IS AN EPIDEMIC?

The emergence of HIV has been referred to as an epidemic. What does this mean? The word *epidemic* is derived from the Greek *epi*—upon—and *demos*—people. The number of new cases of a given disease that occur over a specific period of time is called the incidence rate. When the incidence rate exceeds what is typically expected in a given population in a given location, an epidemic occurs. When an epidemic is restricted to a very limited locale it is often referred to as an outbreak. When it occurs on a global scale, it is called a pandemic. Historically, there have been several influenza pandemics that led to millions of deaths worldwide. These included the Spanish flu pandemic of 1918, the Asian flu of 1957, and the Hong Kong flu of 1968. In 2009, the swine flu (H1N1) was named a pandemic because of its widespread activity across the world.

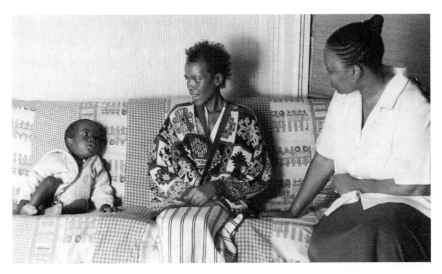

Figure 4.1 AIDS sufferer Purity Khumalo, middle, with her two-year-old HIV-infected son Knowledge in Claremont, South Africa. Nurse Cindi Mshiengu, right, cares for Khumalo at her home as there are simply no resources to care for all AIDS sufferers in state hospitals. (AP/Wide World Photos)

An epidemic often implies rapid and extensive spread of an infection that affects many individuals in an area or a population at the same time. But the term has also been applied to noninfectious societal problems such as obesity and drug addiction. Can you think of ways that these problems are spread?

Thought Box

One historical example of an epidemic is the Black Plague of the Middle Ages. Thousands of people died in Europe because of the spread of a particular bacteria that causes Plague. Can you think of other examples of epidemics? How did they spread? How were they contained?

Infection Models

Imagine that you are a virus that wants to survive. But you need a human host to do so. How would you set up your replication cycle and transmission dynamics so that you could be successfully spread from person to person and continue to exist? It turns out that different viruses answer this question in different ways. Let's look at a few examples to get an idea of how this can be accomplished.

Measles

Although we don't see measles much today, owing to the efficacy of widespread vaccination programs, measles used to be a very common childhood illness. It still occurs in some places in the world, or in people who do not get vaccinated and are exposed to active cases. When an unvaccinated person is exposed to measles, clinical illness often rapidly ensues, usually within two weeks. The measles virus sets up shop in the lining of the mouth, nose, throat, and lungs and causes respiratory illness. It is highly contagious, infecting approximately 90 percent of individuals who are exposed to the virus (through cough, sneeze, or contact with respiratory secretions, for example). The period of infectivity is relatively short, usually ranging from four to nine days. After that, the virus is usually contained by the immune system of an otherwise healthy person and dies out.

HIV

Let's compare measles to the HIV virus. HIV solved the problem of propagating its own infection in a completely different way. Rather than coming on sudden and strong, having a high infectivity rate (90%) and then burning out quickly like measles, HIV has taken somewhat of an opposite approach. While HIV can cause many symptoms when it is first acquired, it then becomes very quiet, often for many years. It has adapted itself to persist for many years within its human host. The actual rate of infectivity is much lower than measles, ranging from approximately $1/10$ to less than $1/1000$ depending on the mechanism of transmission. But because HIV persists for so many years, it can still infect many other people over this longer time course.

Basic Reproductive Rate of Infection

Now let's imagine that you are an unknown virus X, trying to make your stand in the world. What will determine if you will survive in a given population? How many successful infections would it take for you to take a stronghold, and ensure propagation? Scientists have developed a model to study this very question. They reasoned that the factors that influence whether an infection will survive within a population include: the likelihood of infection being transmitted during a contact, the pattern of infectious contacts within the host population (including the number of susceptible people and their interactions with infectious people), and the duration of infectiousness. From this information they created an equation called the Basic reproductive rate of infection (also referred to as Basic Reproductive Number, Basic Reproductive Ratio, or R_0). The R_0 represents the average number of secondary cases a typical single case will cause in a population with no immunity to the disease, in the absence of interventions to control the infection. Here's what the equation looks like:

$$R_0 = \beta \, c \, D$$

where:
* β is the probability of disease transmission per contact,
* c is the number of contacts per unit time, and
* D is the duration of infectiousness

For measles, p is very high but d is very low. For HIV the opposite is true: p is relatively low but d is high.

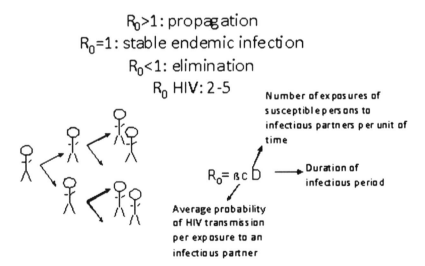

Basic Reproductive Rate

$R_0 > 1$: propagation
$R_0 = 1$: stable endemic infection
$R_0 < 1$: elimination
R_0 HIV: 2-5

Number of exposures of susceptible persons to infectious partners per unit of time

$$R_0 = \beta \, c \, D$$

Duration of infectious period

Average probability of HIV transmission per exposure to an infectious partner

Figure 4.2 The Basic Reproductive Rate of infection is an epidemiologic term that helps predict whether a transmitted illness will propagate or be eliminated.

In order for virus X to survive in a population, the R_0 must be more than 1. This predicts spread of infection in the absence of a specific intervention to stop its propagation. An R_0 that is equal to 1 results in stable "endemic" infection. And an R_0 less than 1 predicts that the disease will die out. Measles has a high R_0, but it was eliminated in some countries by deliberate widespread vaccine campaigns. The relationship between immunization and R_0 can be expressed by a concept called "herd immunity"—the critical threshold of people needed to be vaccinated in order for the disease to be present in such low levels in the population that the risk of infection even in nonimmunized people is dramatically reduced. Mathematically, the proportion of the population that needs to be vaccinated to provide herd immunity and prevent sustained spread of the infection is given by $1 - 1/R_0$. Typically, the higher the R_0, the harder it is to control infection. The HIV R_0 has been estimated to be between 2 and 5. What kinds of ways can you imagine for dropping the HIV R_0 below 1? Now that you have a sense of how R_0 works, you can consider other infections and imagine how they have developed a way to spread. What kind of model do you think is used by tuberculosis? Severe Acute Respiratory Syndrome (or SARS, caused by a coronavirus)? Ebola virus? Chicken pox? Malaria? Others?

EPIDEMIOLOGIC PRINCIPLES: PUTTING IT TOGETHER

We started the chapter by talking about the number of people living with HIV in different parts of the world. The current number of existing cases of a particular disease is often referred to as prevalence of that disease. You can think of this as a snapshot in time. If you looked at the cross-section of a given population at one given instant, how many cases of a particular disease would you find? This concept is in contrast to the number of new cases over a given period of time, which is called incidence, as we discussed earlier. The prevalence of HIV infection in the United States is about one million cases, while estimates of current incidence of HIV infections in the United States are about 56,000 cases per year. Prevalence and incidence are key epidemiologic terms to understand the pattern of diseases. You can also think about these words as they apply to other problems: How would you describe the prevalence of teen pregnancy compared to the incidence of teen pregnancy? What other examples can you think of?

SUMMARY

HIV affects nearly every country of the world, but the highest burden by far is in sub-Saharan Africa, where an estimated 22–23 million cases of the globally

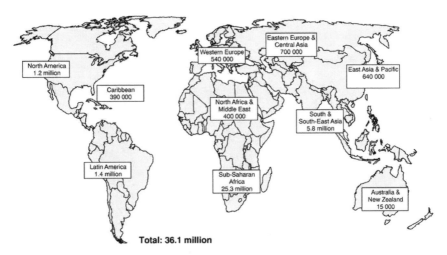

Figure 4.3 Estimated global prevalence of HIV by approximate number of cases per geographic region. (World Health Organization 2008)

estimated 34 million cases have occurred. Although the death rate has declined after the introduction of effective HIV treatment, the number of new cases in the United States—estimated at about 56,000 per year—has remained distressingly unchanged. This suggests that prevention strategies are not effective enough. Increased outreach and educational programs are needed to decrease high-risk behaviors and prevent further spread of the epidemic. A disease becomes an epidemic when the number of new infections over a given period of time—the incidence rate—exceeds what is typically expected in a given population in a given location. The basic reproductive rate is an equation that can be used to estimate whether a given infection will propagate, stay stable, or be eradicated. Prevalence (the number of infections in a given location at a particular snapshot of time) and the incidence of infection are key epidemiologic terms that can help describe a particular disease.

5

HIV Transmission

Courtney L. McMickens, MD, MPH

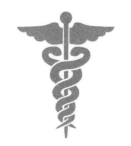

This chapter reviews how HIV is spread, specific groups at higher risk for infection, and strategies for prevention. We will also take a look around the world and explore some of the barriers several countries have faced in addressing the spread of HIV. We will focus on the following issues:

- How is HIV transmitted from one person to another?
- Which groups of people are at particularly high risk for HIV infection?
- What is the relationship between HIV and other sexually transmitted diseases?
- What is the relative risk of transmission during different stages of HIV infection?
- How is HIV transmitted from mother to child?
- What can we learn from case studies of HIV transmission?
  - China: blood market
  - India: truck routes
  - Africa: a lack of political willpower
- How can transmission be prevented?
  - Education

- Screening
- Behavioral changes

HOW IS HIV TRANSMITTED?

HIV is transmitted through exposure to infected blood or bodily fluids, such as semen, genital secretions, and breast milk. Blood or fluid exchange can be the result of activities such as sexual intercourse, intravenous drug use, or transfusion of contaminated blood or blood products. Transfusion of blood or blood products once carried the highest risk of transmission, with a nearly universal 100 percent risk of transmission if an individual was transfused with infected blood or blood products. However, following the availability of a method for detecting HIV in the blood in 1985, use of this test to screen donated blood products for HIV in many countries around the world dramatically reduced this statistic. Today, the risk of HIV transmission from a blood transfusion in the United States has dropped to about 1:1,000,000. Some of the higher risks of HIV transmission can result from a contaminated needle stick (from a source patient with infected blood), sharing needles, and certain sexual practices, particularly between men who have sex with men (MSM).

The relative risk of transmission through sexual contact depends on the nature of the sexual activity as well as the relative infectiousness of the HIV-positive sexual partner (which is most closely correlated with the level of virus in the blood). However, the disease is quite complex, with several other factors that also affect the rate of transmission. These factors include viral subtype, coinfection with sexually transmitted diseases, stage of HIV infection, an individual's innate susceptibility to HIV infection, and amount of virus in genital secretions. In general, receptive anal intercourse with an infected person is considered to carry the highest risk of sexual transmission, followed by vaginal intercourse, and then receptive oral sex with ejaculation (which is much lower risk unless there are open sores or cuts in the mouth).

Some experts refer to the risk of HIV transmission from sexual intercourse as a "low probability, but high stakes" event. This means that although transmission does not necessarily happen every time there is an exposure, the consequences of becoming infected are so significant and lifelong that making sure to take appropriate preventive measures is extremely important and worthwhile.

HIV may also be transmitted from mother to child during pregnancy, delivery, and breast feeding. Studies have shown that HIV can be transmitted to the fetus in the first and second trimester, but the highest rate of transmission from mother to child occurs during labor and delivery, also known as the intrapartum period. Use of antiretroviral medication and other protective interventions during pregnancy, such as delivery by Caesarian section when necessary, has greatly decreased the transmission of HIV infection to the infant. These risk reduction methods will be further discussed later in this chapter.

Despite mass educational campaigns, there continues to be misconception regarding the mechanisms of HIV transmission. There is no evidence to suggest that HIV can be transmitted by casual touch of intact skin or closed-mouth kissing in the absence of open sores. There is also no evidence that HIV can be transmitted from exposure to tears or sweat of an infected individual. HIV also cannot be transmitted through the air, water, or insects. Contact in the work place, including through food preparation, does not increase the risk of HIV transmission when recommended standards and practices of personal hygiene

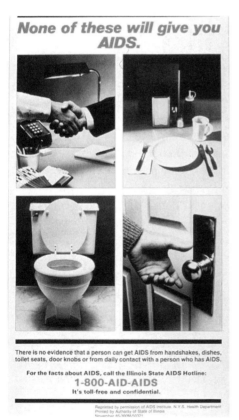

Figure 5.1 AIDS awareness poster visually refutes myths about how HIV/AIDS is contracted. In the early years after the disease emerged in the United States, there was widespread ignorance and panic regarding the virus. (National Library of Medicine)

and food sanitation are followed. HIV is also not transmitted by shared use of water fountains. Though the risk is low, there is a potential for transmission with open-mouth or "French kissing," if there are mouth sores or lacerations present.

If one is living with someone who is HIV positive, transmission within households is rare and can be avoided with the use of precautionary measures. These measures include: wearing gloves when handling blood-containing fluids, covering any open sores or cuts on the HIV-positive person with bandages, hand-washing regularly, avoiding the sharing of razors and toothbrushes, and immediately disposing of needles such as diabetic syringes or other sharp instruments properly into puncture-proof containers.

AT-RISK GROUPS

It is estimated that there were approximately 56,300 new cases of HIV in the United States in 2006. About half of the newly diagnosed cases of HIV were among individuals who engaged in male-to-male sexual contact. Another 31 percent of the newly diagnosed cases of HIV were attributed to heterosexual contact, and about 12 percent were attributed to injection drug use (see Figure 5.2). Injection drug use not only includes intravenous drug use, but it also includes subdermal and intramuscular injections, known as "skin-popping" and "muscling," respectively. Individuals who engage in receptive anal intercourse, injection drug use, and unprotected sex with multiple partners are considered to be at the highest risks of contracting HIV. In the United States, men who have sex with men (or MSM) represents the at-risk group with the highest overall percent of HIV infections.

Over the past 20 years, the number of cases among heterosexual women has increased dramatically. Data also show that HIV and AIDS disproportionally affect minority populations, with African Americans accounting for nearly half of the new HIV cases in 2006. The prevalence rate for Hispanic/Latino men (883 per 100,000) was more than two times the rate for white men (395 per100,000), while the prevalence rate for Hispanic/Latino women (263 per 100,000) was four times the rate for white women (63 per 100,000). Young adults are also disproportionately affected, with the majority of new AIDS cases occurring among age groups 25–34 and 35–44.

Recently there has been an increase in HIV cases among MSM. Risk factors that may be contributing to this recent increase in transmission include an increased participation in unprotected sex, lack of knowledge regarding partner's status, and an increase in other sexually transmitted diseases, which can increase the risk of HIV transmission. Research also suggests that the prevalence of drug

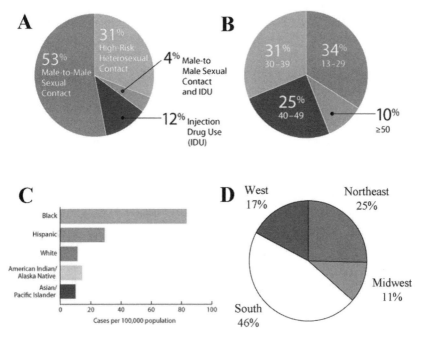

Figure 5.2 Relative distribution of HIV infections in the United States, 2006 (A-C) and 2007 (D). A: Estimated distribution of new U.S. HIV infections in 2006 by transmission categories. B: Estimated distribution of new U.S. HIV infections by age group. C: Estimated rates of new U.S. HIV infections by race and ethnicity. D: Distribution of AIDS diagnoses in 2007 by U.S. region. (Centers for Disease Control)

and alcohol use within the MSM community may play a role in sexual decision making and subsequent risk taking.

Treatment for HIV/AIDS has also been hypothesized to play a role in the pattern of transmission in two major ways. First, the success of antiretroviral medication has prolonged and improved the quality of life for individuals with HIV. However, the medication does not cure the disease, so there is theoretically a lifelong risk of transmission for the partners of treated HIV-positive individuals. Second, some studies suggest that the success of antiretroviral medications has decreased the fear of imminent death and negative views associated with HIV, and therefore, individual are less cautious in their sexual encounters.

For ethnic and racial minority groups, the burden of HIV/AIDS is great at each stage of the disease. African Americans make up 13 percent of the population in the United States and accounted for 49 percent of the new cases of HIV in the United States in 2006. Hispanic/Latino Americans make up 15 percent of the population in the United States and accounted for 17 percent of the new HIV cases in 2006. Sixty-one percent of the individuals under the age of 25 diagnosed with HIV between 2001 and 2005 were African American.

Hispanics/Latinos have the second-highest rate of infection following African Americans, making AIDS the fourth leading cause of death among Hispanics/Latinos ages 35–44. The risk factors for African Americans and Hispanic/Latino Americans are similar to those identified among MSM. These include high prevalence of unprotected sex, drug use, and other coexisting sexually transmitted infections. Additionally, cultural and socioeconomic factors must be taken into account. According to the Centers for Disease Control, nearly one in four African American and nearly one in five Hispanic/Latino American lives in poverty. Studies have found a significant association between higher HIV rates and poverty. Stigma surrounding HIV within minority communities impedes efforts to have frank conversations regarding transmission and prevention of disease. Immigration may also pose challenges to prevention strategies such as regular screening and testing.

Other groups who are at risk of becoming infected with HIV include health-care workers, sexual partners of individuals who engage in risky sexual behavior or injection drug use, and victims of unwanted sexual contact. Health-care workers are at risk of occupational transmission of HIV due to accidental needle sticks for example; however, this risk is very small when universal precautions are used while caring for patients and handling contaminated material.

If a health-care worker is exposed to HIV, the individual should be tested for HIV and treated with antiretroviral therapy immediately using a strategy called post-exposure prophylaxis (or PEP), which can significantly decrease the risk of transmission from the exposure. Individuals who have sexual contact with those in high-risk groups are considered to be at high risk for HIV transmission. Risk reduction techniques include abstinence, or the use of safer sex practices, such as latex condoms and/or other barrier protection. Regular testing for HIV is recommended in the latter scenario, since the protection afforded is not 100 percent, and breeches of protection can occur (such as condom rupture or other condom accidents). Some experts advocate the role of antiretroviral therapy in individuals who are HIV positive as a preventive measure, since lowering the viral load decreases the likelihood of transmission. And new studies are exploring the use of antiretroviral medications before exposure to HIV (so-called pre-exposure prophylasxis, or PrEP) as a public health strategy to prevent transmission. What do you think about this approach?

HIV AND OTHER SEXUALLY TRANSMITTED INFECTIONS

Having unprotected sexual intercourse not only puts one at risk for acquiring HIV, but it also puts an individual at risk for other sexually transmitted infections (STIs). These STIs (such as herpes, syphilis, gonorrhea, chlamydia, and others) are far more common than HIV and may increase the risk of HIV transmission. Sexually transmitted infections can be divided into ulcerative and nonulcerative STIs. Common ulcerative diseases include herpes, syphilis, and chancroid. These STIs cause ulcers that promote infectivity in two ways: (1) for an HIV negative partner with an ulcerative STI, there is increased risk of exposure to the virus resulting from a breech in the skin at the site of the ulcer; and (2) for an HIV-positive partner with an ulcerative STI, there is an increased concentration of HIV at the site of the ulcer because of accelerated replication of virus-containing cells at this site of injury, increasing the likelihood of transmission.

Nonulcerative STIs such as trichomonas, chlamydia, and gonorrhea also increase the risk of HIV transmission. Studies suggest that the inflammatory state associated with STIs may result in an increased concentration of the virus in seminal fluid and vaginal secretions, because of an increased number of lymphocytes and monocytes that are called in by the immune system, which is activated by the STI. Men infected with both gonorrhea and HIV are more than twice as likely to have HIV in their genital secretions at a concentration up to 10 times higher compared to men infected with HIV alone. Therefore, screening, prevention, and treatment of other STIs is critical to preventing the transmission of HIV. Also, because of the shared mechanism of transmission, a diagnosis of an STI should prompt consideration of testing for HIV, and vice versa.

RELATIVE RISK OF HIV TRANSMISSION DURING DIFFERENT STAGES OF HIV INFECTION

HIV infection can be divided into three general stages—acute (also sometimes referred to as primary), latent (also known as the asymptomatic stage), and late (or advanced). The rate of transmission varies between each stage, with highest infectiousness in the primary stage, followed by the late stage.

The acute or primary stage refers to the first few weeks of infection. This stage is characterized by an acute clinical syndrome lasting two to six weeks after infection, in which an individual may experience fever, sore throat, swollen lymph nodes, joint pain, nausea, loss of appetite, and other flu-like symptoms. During this time the HIV virus replicates rapidly while the body mounts an immune response. There is a transient period of extremely high infectiousness due to the extremely high levels of virus in the blood. One study estimates that the risk of transmission within the first few weeks of infection is eight to ten times higher in the acute stage when compare to the asymptomatic stage. It is estimated that up to a half of newly transmitted cases of HIV occur during the primary stage of the disease.

Following the acute phase of infection, gradually the body gains the ability to defend itself, and the symptoms subside. The number of CD4 cells, the specific type of white blood cell that HIV infects, returns to normal or near-normal levels in the majority of cases, and individuals enter the asymptomatic or latent stage of the disease, which can last several years untreated. During this stage HIV viral replication is ongoing, and the disease progresses. Progression and infectiousness depend on the levels of HIV virus in the blood, the subtype of HIV, and host factors that affect the immune response to HIV, and therefore they vary from case to case. Eventually, there is a decline in the body's immune system to a level in which the body is no longer able to protect itself against certain illnesses.

The third stage of HIV is defined by a low CD4 count, opportunistic infections, and other illnesses. The diagnosis of acquired immunodeficiency syndrome (AIDS) is determined by these factors and marks the final stage of the disease, which can vary in length. Infectiousness rises again in the late stage due to high viral concentrations in the blood. The risk of transmission within two years of death has been estimated to be four to eight times higher in the late stage when compared to the asymptomatic stage.

PREGNANCY

HIV can be transmitted from an infected mother to her fetus during pregnancy, delivery, or by breastfeeding. This is known as perinatal, or mother-to-child transmission. The highest rate of transmission occurs in the intrapartum period—the stage that includes labor and delivery—though transmission can take place as early as the first trimester and also after delivery. Based on studies done in Rwanda and Zaire, the risks of transmission from an HIV-positive mother to her child, in the absence of any treatment, have been estimated to be as high as 23–30 percent during pregnancy, 50–65 percent during labor and delivery, and 12–20 percent as a result of breastfeeding. In the U.S. the overall risk of transmitting HIV from a positive mother to her baby is estimated at approximately 15–30 percent i the absence of treatment.

Factors that influence transmission of HIV from mother to fetus/infant include access to and adequacy of prenatal care, general health of the mother, stage of disease, HIV screening, and availability of antiretroviral treatment. The use of antiretroviral therapy to treat HIV-positive mothers and their infants has made a dramatic difference in the outcomes for these families. In 1994, a study, known as the PACTG 076 study, examined the use of the antiretroviral medication zidovudine (also known as AZT) in women and their babies and showed that treatment of an infected mother beginning in the second trimester through delivery, along with treatment of the newborn for six weeks, resulted in a relative reduction of HIV transmission by 67.5 percent.

The PACTG 076 study was followed by another study known as the HIV-NET 012 study. In the HIVNET study investigators compared the effectiveness of preventing maternal-to-fetal transmission with a very short course of the antiretroviral medication nevirapine compared to a short course of zidovudine. Nevirapine or zidovudine was given to HIV-positive mothers at the beginning of labor. One dose of nevirapine was given to the nevirapine group of infants within 72 hours of life, and zidovudine was given to the zidovudine group of infants for seven days. In this landmark study, two doses of nevirapine—one pill given to the mother at onset of labor, and one given to the baby 72 hours after birth—lowered the risk of HIV transmission by nearly 50 percent. The results of this study were especially meaningful for developing countries with limited resources and limited ability to provide the seven-to-eight month course of zidovudine outlined in the PACTG study.

Currently in the United States, the rate of mother-to-child transmission is less than 1 percent with the use of combination antiretroviral therapy. Treatment and regular testing, caesarean section for mothers with unsuppressed viral loads, and avoidance of breastfeeding when feasible (i.e., clean water and affordable formula are available) are methods that have aided in the reduction of transmission.

In spite of these efforts and successes, there are still an estimated 100–200 infants infected with HIV in the United States annually. The mother's lack of awareness of her HIV status is the major factor that has been noted as a barrier to prevention. Overall, it is estimated that approximately 25 percent of all people with HIV are unaware of their status, pregnant women included in this group. In 2002, a study of 748 women revealed that 31 percent had never been tested for HIV during their prior pregnancy. The rate of HIV testing among pregnant women, who are at risk by definition, varies from state to state.

In 2006, the Center for Disease Control set forth a recommendation for routine "opt-out" HIV screening. This strategy consists of routine testing of all pregnant women in the first trimester and repeat testing in the third trimester for those who meet high-risk criteria, unless the woman specifically declines testing. The campaign with the slogan "One Test. Two Lives" provides HIV prevention-related information for health-care providers and patients. Early identification of women who are HIV-positive during pregnancy allows more rapid initiation of HIV-specific care, and therefore decreased risk of transmission to the infant. Treatment guidelines in the U.S. support treatment of HIV-positive women regardless of their CD4 count for this reason. We'll learn more about treatment in chapter 7.

Thought Box

What do you think: Should an "opt-out" testing policy be implemented for all individuals over the age of 16?

CASE STUDIES

The HIV/AIDS epidemic has affected many cultures throughout the world. Each country has faced its own challenges in reducing the transmission of HIV. In some countries, social and cultural norms, including sexual practices, stigma, and poverty, have facilitated the spread of HIV. Three case examples that have contributed to the transmission of HIV around the world are presented here. This is by no means a complete list, but is meant to give you a general sense of the kinds of issues that can contribute to the challenges of controlling HIV transmission.

China

Since the beginning of the HIV/AIDS epidemic, countries around the world, including the United States, have faced the issue of a contaminated blood supply. The availability of a test to detect HIV in the blood in 1985 greatly improved the ability to keep the blood supply clean. Many countries quickly employed testing strategies once they became available, investigated the sources of contamination and regulated blood collection and distribution in the 1980s to clean up their blood supply. But in the mid-1990s an increase in the incidence of HIV was noted in a rural population in China. Villagers began to come to medical attention after they were infected with HIV—a problem that was ultimately tracked back to their local blood collection center.

The scarcity of donated blood and pervasive poverty in the countryside of China set up a "perfect storm": businessmen, known as "blood heads," directed the illegal collection of blood and plasma. Habitants of rural villages in the Henan Province were especially hard hit. The "blood heads" traveled throughout the countryside of the Henan Province, offering monetary compensation for blood donations. The blood was then pooled, and the plasma was separated and packaged. The remaining blood products, now pooled and untested for HIV, were transfused back into each seller, placing him at the greatest risk of HIV infection.

Thought Box

Other groups have historically been at extremely high risk of HIV infection because of pooled blood products from many donors who were not tested for HIV. Can you remember another such group discussed in chapter 1?

It is estimated that illegal blood trade was responsible for six to ten percent of the 600,000 new cases of HIV in China during the early 1990s. In 1997, the Chinese government addressed the Henan blood market scandal by establishing regulatory procedures for blood collection and penalties for violations. In 1999, the Blood Donation Law, which mandated testing of blood donations, was passed; however, the feasibility of placing facilities in the rural regions of China was questioned because of both the remote location and the fact that extreme poverty served as an ongoing incentive for villagers to participate in illegal blood donation.

Since the 1990s, China has made great progress in the effort to clean up the blood supply, destroying HIV-positive stockpiles, closing hundreds of collection stations, and making several arrests. The Chinese Ministry of Health reports that a demand for blood and blood products, coupled with the profitability of blood sales, sustains some illegal blood market activity. As of 2007, it is estimated that blood sales were the source of up to 20 percent of the Chinese blood supply. China continues to fight the illegal blood market with the implementation of new and more comprehensive regulation of blood collection and testing.

India

The first case of HIV in India was found in Chennai, Tamil Nadu, in 1986. Twenty years later, in 2006, there were an estimated 5.7 million individuals living with HIV in India. Sexual transmission accounted for more than 85 percent of HIV infections. High-risk groups include truck drivers, injection drug users, those with sexually transmitted infections, and female sex workers. Prevalence among these groups was estimated to be 10–20 percent.

India's four major cities, New Delhi, Mumbai, Chennai, and Kolkata, are along an express highway, known as the Golden Quadrilateral, which is frequently traveled by long-distance truckers. The prevalence of HIV along the Golden Quadrilateral is greater than 5 percent, compared to a national prevalence of 0.5–1.5 percent. Clients of sex workers along the Golden Quadrilateral, especially truck drivers, are believed to play a significant role in the spread of HIV in India. The truckers engage in activities with a sex worker and then return home to their partners after weeks to months on the road. The prevalence of HIV in commercial sex workers became increasingly high, resulting in transmissions to truckers, who then placed their partners at home at risk of becoming infected. Remember that the risk of infection is highest by up to 10 times at the earliest stages of infection, just when a trucker who acquired HIV infection on the road would be returning home.

At one treatment facility in Chennai, a quarter of those newly diagnosed with HIV are housewives. There has been a countrywide attempt to increase condom use; however, societal beliefs that condom use promotes promiscuity have been a challenge to this prevention strategy.

Africa

Africa has faced a major battle against the HIV epidemic, particularly in sub-Saharan Africa, which shoulders the greatest burden of this disease. The HIV prevalence in the country of South Africa is approximately 18.8 percent, and in 2005, it is estimated that there were almost 900 deaths per day from AIDS. By the late 1990s the use of antiretroviral medications to prevent mother-to-child transmission was well established. However, not all political leaders readily accepted this method of prevention. In 1999, the president of South Africa, Thabo Mbeki, announced that the South African government would not fund the antiretroviral therapy for HIV-positive mothers because the drugs were toxic. The South African government made many efforts to deny that HIV caused AIDS and attempted to promote nutrition and vitamins as treatments. A study estimating the lost benefit of this decision examined the number of deaths from 2000 to 2005. The investigator estimated that there were 60,000 newly infected babies each year. Without antiretroviral therapy, the excess infections totaled 35,532, which was an approximate loss of 1.6 million person-years. Though programs for the distribution of antiretrovirals were numerous in South Africa in 2009, the challenge of correcting some ongoing inaccurate health messages can leave the population ill-informed and at risk for further spread of HIV.

PREVENTION

Much work has been done to develop a vaccine for HIV, but as of 2011, this has proven unsuccessful. Therefore, the mainstay of prevention remains education regarding HIV and safer sexual practices, encouraging behavioral change, and regular testing.

Education

The most essential weapon against the transmission of HIV currently is education. Programs informing the population about risk factors, testing, and HIV disease progression play a vital role in awareness, destigmatization, and prevention. Several studies have shown that comprehensive sex education and HIV prevention programs decrease high-risk activity and/or delay initiation of sexual activity. Because adolescents and young adults made up 16 percent of newly diagnosed cases of HIV in 2006, the importance of early educational programs is emphasized by the public health community. Primary care doctors should obtain a sexual history from all patients and review the risk factors for becoming infected with HIV as well as other STIs. Some school-based prevention programs have also been shown to be effective.

Behavioral Changes

Behavior modification is very important in the prevention of HIV transmission. The only method of absolutely preventing sexual transmission of HIV is abstinence. For those who are not abstinent, safer sexual practices must be adopted to prevent transmission. These practices include involvement in a monogamous relationship, condom use, and/or avoiding specific high-risk activities. Recent data suggest that male circumcision can also reduce HIV transmission. Individuals are encouraged to participate in monogamous sexual relationships and to have honest discussions with their partners about HIV status and testing. Use of latex condoms decreases the transmission of HIV dramatically, though it is not 100 percent effective. Condom failure is usually the result of breakage or improper use. Water-based lubricants can help avoid some condom failures. Natural skin condoms, such as lamb skin, and petroleum-based lubricants are generally less effective.

The cessation of injection drug use is the most effective method to decrease transmission from sharing of needles. Efforts to reduce risk and support individuals with drug problems include expanded substance abuse treatment programs. Individuals who continue to use are encouraged to avoid sharing needles and other drug paraphernalia, such as cookers and spoons. While controversial, some states have implemented needle exchange programs to replace used needles with new sterile ones. Some opponents argue that providing clean needles condones intravenous drug use and could increase this behavior. However, so far needle-exchange programs have resulted in a decrease in the transmission of HIV without increasing the prevalence of intravenous drug use.

Thought Box

What do you think: is clean needle exchange a good prevention strategy for HIV infection? Why or why not?

Screening

It is estimated that about 25 percent of those infected with HIV in the United States are unaware of their status and hence place others at risk of infection. Therefore, in 2006 the Centers of Disease Control has recommended that all adults should be routinely tested in a new strategy called universal screening. Recommendations include informed testing for individuals between the ages of 13 and 64 without requiring written consent. In the CDC strategy, in addition to obtaining a detailed sexual history and risk assessment, physicians are expected to discuss the meaning of a positive test prior to testing, and the individual reserves the right to opt out of testing. This type of routine testing program could decrease transmission by behavioral modification and reduce disease progression through early diagnosis and intervention. Studies have shown that HIV-positive individuals who are aware of their status decrease their participation in high-risk behaviors. Detection of HIV at an earlier stage would allow for early intervention, decreased viral load, and decreased transmission. It is also thought that routine testing could destigmatize HIV testing and infection. However, implementation of the CDC recommendations has been slow because many state laws still require full informed consent before testing mandating more time and resources.

Recall from chapter 1 that testing for HIV involves two steps—initial screening and confirmatory testing. The most common testing method used for initial screening in the United States is the enzyme-linked immuno-sorbent assay (ELISA), also called the enzyme immunoassay (EIA), which is very sensitive test that is performed on a blood sample. A positive test must be confirmed by a second, more specific, test known as a western blot. Both of these tests detect antibodies that are made by the body to respond to HIV infection, but the western blot can differentiate antibodies specific to HIV from others that may have falsely resulted in a positive ELISA. If the ELISA test is negative, testing should be repeated in six months for individuals with a history of HIV risk factors, due to the possibility of a false negative during the "window period" of new infection, which can range from weeks to months. During the window period, the HIV test is negative because it takes the body weeks or months to develop anti-HIV antibodies. During this time, an HIV viral load is necessary to detect early infection. This test, if positive, should be confirmed with antibody testing.

SUMMARY

HIV is a virus that is today most commonly transmitted through sexual intercourse, injectable drug use, and from mother-to-fetus. The virus, which attacks the body's immune system, can be found in blood, blood products, bodily fluid, and body tissue. Activities like engaging in unprotected sex or sharing needles places one at greater risk for infection. Education and awareness, regular testing, the use of condoms, and treatment of other STIs are important preventative methods against the transmission of HIV. The use of antiretroviral therapy has dramatically decreased the rates of transmission to infants of HIV-positive mothers. Until there is a vaccine for HIV, education, behavior modification, and screening continue to be the mainstay of prevention.

6

How Does HIV Affect the Body?

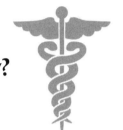

Sigall K. Bell, MD

*This chapter discusses the natural history of HIV infection from the time of initial in-
fection to the development of severe immunodeficiency, opportunistic infections, and
AIDS. In this chapter we will focus on:*

- What are the early events in the body following acquisition of HIV?
- What is the body's initial immune response to HIV?
- What is the "acute retroviral syndrome"?
- What is the typical timeline from infection to AIDS?
- What are the phases of HIV infection?
- What are the symptoms and signs of advanced HIV infection?
- What are opportunistic infections?
- What is antibiotic prophylaxis and how is it used?
- What are some nonopportunistic complications of HIV?
- What are some important interactions of HIV with other coinfections?
  - HIV and hepatitis
  - HIV and tuberculosis
  - HIV and syphilis

ACQUISITION OF HIV AND EARLY EVENTS

HIV is primarily acquired through exposure to blood or bodily fluids containing the virus. Common modes of acquisition include sexual intercourse, intravenous drug use, transfusion with contaminated blood or blood products, or transmission from mother to child during pregnancy, delivery, or breast feeding. A blood test for HIV became available in 1985, after which the blood supply was screened for evidence of this virus. Prior to this time, however, some people requiring transfusions acquired the virus from a contaminated blood supply. This is particularly true of hemophiliacs, or individuals with blood disorders, who required large amounts of transfusions. In some developing countries, contaminated blood or blood products is still a problem.

When HIV first enters the body it is recognized by particular cells whose job it is to detect foreign particles such as viruses, using specialized receptors on their cell surface. HIV is then transported to local lymph nodes, where it can multiply. The virus enters the bloodstream within days to weeks and can then spread to every part of the body. At this point it undergoes rapid replication, producing up to 10 billion virus particles per day. A blood test called the viral load test can

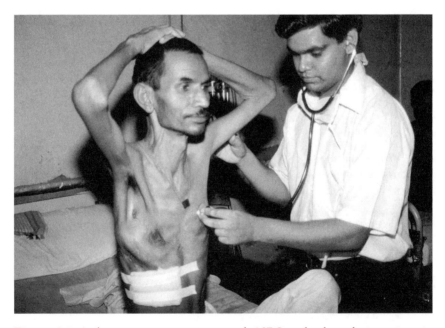

Figure 6.1 A doctor examines a suspected AIDS and tuberculosis patient in New Delhi in 2002. (Pallava Bagla/Cobis Sygma)

measure the amount of virus in the blood. During the earliest stage of infection (also called acute infection or primary infection), the viral load is the highest it will ever be during the course of infection over many years; usually greater than one million copies of virus per milliliter of blood.

THE BODY'S IMMUNE RESPONSE TO HIV

Remember that the body responds to the newly recognized HIV infection by mobilizing many of its immune defenses. The very first encounter that the body has with HIV during acute HIV infection is a highly dynamic time, when the body and the virus are at battle, as the human host attempts to control the virus. However, the virus is clever and fast and usually evades host control. During the battle, activation of the immune system results in the release of many important cell-signaling chemicals called cytokines. Cytokines help to further activate the immune system, but they can also cause symptoms like fever and body aches.

Over time, the body develops antibodies directed at HIV, to try to control spread of the infection. However, this can take weeks to months. The blood test for HIV relies on the presence of this antibody. This means that during the period of acute HIV infection, the test may be falsely negative. Therefore diagnosis during this early time requires a viral load test in addition to the HIV antibody test. If the HIV antibody result is negative or equivocal in someone suspected to have new HIV infection, it should be repeated about six weeks later to confirm the formation of a positive antibody. Despite the presence of antibody later in infection, most people cannot maintain control of the virus without medication.

THE ACUTE RETROVIRAL SYNDROME:
SYMPTOMS AND SIGNS OF NEW INFECTION

Most people develop some symptoms during the period of acute HIV infection. Common symptoms include fever, chills, sweats, sore throat, body aches, nausea, vomiting, diarrhea, and headache (see Table 6.1). The group of symptoms and signs are often collectively called the acute retroviral syndrome, since HIV is a type of retrovirus. A few laboratory tests (like white blood cell count, platelet count, or liver function tests) may also be abnormal during this time, although these findings are not in and of themselves diagnostic of HIV. Whether the symptoms and signs of acute HIV infection are due to direct effects of the virus itself or due to the "cytokine storm" as the host immune system is activated is not known. Both factors likely contribute to the early symptoms. It is estimated that 50–90 percent of people develop symptoms, but these may range from very

Table 6.1 Common Signs and Symptoms of Acute HIV Infection

Common Clinical Findings	Common Laboratory Findings
Fever	Low white blood cell count
Sore throat	Low platelet count
Swollen glands	Elevated liver function tests
Rash	Low CD4 count
Muscle aches	High viral load
Joint pain	
Night sweats	
Stomach ache	
Vomiting	
Diarrhea	
Headache	
Stiff neck	
Loss of appetite	
Weight loss	
Oral or genital ulcers	

mild to very severe, sometimes requiring hospitalization. Because the symptoms are so similar to the common cold or flu, they often go unrecognized as acute HIV infection, delaying the diagnosis, often for many years.

TIMELINE FROM INFECTION TO AIDS

The phase of acute HIV infection is over, by definition, when an HIV antibody appears. In some people this can happen as early as two weeks; in others it can take six months. Once the antibody forms, the individual enters the period of early infection, which lasts for the first 6 to 12 months. During this time, the body and the virus reach a steady state, or equilibrium (after weeks or months of battle), where viral replication is held in check at some more or less constant level. This can range anywhere from undetectable levels of virus in the blood to very high levels like >100,000 copies/mL. The steady state is called the viral set point, and this is believed to be predictive of disease progression. Individuals with a very low viral set point generally have slower progression of HIV disease. Individuals with a high viral set point often progress more rapidly.

At this point, the infection enters a quiet phase (sometimes also called the period of latency), because even though virus continues to replicate, the human host often does not have any symptoms. If the diagnosis was not made during the period of acute HIV infection (as it is often not since symptoms at that time are not specific and may be thought to be a simple flu-like illness), the person may not have any knowledge or suspicion that they are infected. This is problematic because such persons may go on to infect other people.

Because the risk of transmission to others is correlated with the degree of viral load, transmission is especially high during acute infection, when the level of virus in the blood and bodily fluids is so extraordinarily high. In fact, studies have shown that the rate of transmission during this early phase may be 10 times higher than in other stages of infection, and that up to 50 percent of all transmission events occur during acute infection.

The latency period of HIV infection can last for months to years, depending on the rate of disease progression. On average, it usually lasts about 5 to 10 years. Again, during this time, the individual is asymptomatic from the HIV perspective. However, as HIV infects and destroys CD4 T lymphocyte cells, the number of these cells slowly drops, and the human host becomes more and more immunosuppressed. When the CD4 cell count falls below 200 cells/μL, the individual

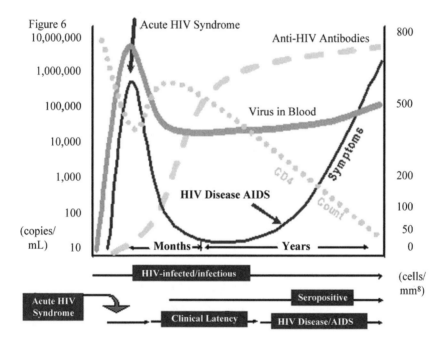

Figure 6.2 Schematic diagram of changes in HIV viral load, CD4 cell count, HIV antibody status, and clinical symptoms over time in an untreated individual. Acute HIV is typically a symptomatic period occurring after infection and before formation of HIV antibody, when the viral load is very high. AIDS occurs when the CD4 count declines to or below 200. (Courtesy of Jon Fuller, MD)

is classified as having AIDS. During acute HIV infection there is a transient dip in the CD4 count, followed by a restoration to near normal values (of about 500–1200 cells/μL). Subsequently, the CD4 count declines by about 100 cells per year on average, resulting in a diagnosis of AIDS over about 5 to 10 years if left untreated. In some people this decline can be more rapid.

SYMPTOMS OF ADVANCED HIV DISEASE AND AIDS

The symptoms of more advanced HIV infection or AIDS are due to a weakened immune system. At this point, individuals are susceptible to many infections and complications. Because they lack strong immune response, persons with advanced disease can get sick from illnesses that most people with intact immune systems can fight off. These include so-called opportunistic infections like PCP (pneumocystis pneumonia), cryptococcus, MAI (mycobacteria avium intracellulare), and reactivation of prior toxoplasmosis or cytomegalovirus infections.

EXAMPLES OF SOME OPPORTUNISTIC INFECTIONS

PCP

Pneumocystis pneumonia is a very common opportunistic infection in patients with HIV. You'll recall it was one of the first infections that was recognized in "clusters" when HIV was first recognized (although not yet named!) in 1981. PCP causes a diffuse pneumonia that most commonly looks like scattered infiltrates in what is called an "interstitial" pattern on a chest X-ray. This is in contrast to usual community-acquired bacterial pneumonias that often show more of a consolidated "lobar" pattern. Patients with PCP have a subacute course, typically evolving over days to weeks. The characteristic finding is a low oxygen saturation—a test that doctors can perform by putting a probe on the patient's finger—that gets even worse with exertion, for example when the patient walks.

PCP is most commonly seen when the CD4 count falls below 200 cells/μL. For this reason, doctors recommend a medicine to prevent PCP infection in patients who have a CD4 count that falls below this threshold. The most commonly used antibiotic is trimethoprim-sulfamethoxasole (commonly called Bactrim). This strategy is called antibiotic prophylaxis—a term that implies that the patient is treated ahead of time, *before* the infection occurs, to *prevent* the onset of illness.

MAI

MAI is a type of mycobacterial infection. Mycobacteria are a class of organisms that have a waxy component to their cell wall, including tuberculosis (TB), but MAI is a nontuberculous mycobacteria. It causes a different range of symptoms than TB, including abdominal pain, diarrhea, weight loss, fever, and swollen glands. MAI can also invade the bone marrow and result in a drop in the blood cell counts (including red blood cells, white blood cells, and platelets). MAI can appear in disseminated form, which means it can travel to many parts of the body at once. MAI is most commonly seen in very advanced AIDS, when the CD4 count is less than 50 cells/µL.

Doctors also recommend prophylactic antibiotics for MAI that should be initiated when the CD4 count falls below 50 cells/µL. This is most commonly accomplished using a medicine called azithromycin, which can be taken in one big dose, once a week.

Toxoplasmosis

Cerebral toxoplasmosis is an example of a reactivation infection that causes—as the name implies—an infection in the brain. Reactivation means that the patient already has been exposed to toxoplasmosis, but the lower immunity with more advanced AIDS allows the old infection to rekindle. This is similar in principle to the reactivation of the varicella zoster virus causing shingles that we discussed in chapter 2; however, a more profound level of immunosuppression is usually required to reactivate toxoplasmosis. Toxoplasma are very common organisms that many of us are exposed to by the time we become adults. It is particularly common in cats and can be transmitted by changing cat litter, for example, but can also be acquired from other sources in the environment. Many healthy people never know that they were exposed to toxoplasma, because the immune system controls the infection effectively and we may never experience symptoms. We can test to see if we have ever been exposed to toxoplasma by looking for an antibody to it in the blood. If the antibody is present in a person with HIV, they are then at risk for reactivation of toxoplasmosis, and this most commonly occurs in the brain. If the antibody is not already present, then patients with HIV should be particularly careful not to acquire new (or primary) toxoplasma infection. This means they should avoid changing cat litter if possible, for example, or wear gloves and wash their hands carefully, if they must do this task.

Toxoplasma are parasites that typically cause several lesions in the brain. Each lesion is characteristically surrounded by inflammation that looks like a bright, or "enhancing" ring on CAT scan imaging of the head. Patients who have toxoplasmosis can develop seizures, a change in mental status or loss of consciousness, or sudden onset of weakness or abnormal sensation in certain parts of their body—appearing as though they have had a stroke. They can also have cranial nerve deficits, resulting in problems with vision or facial nerve function, for example. The particular symptoms seen in any given individual depend on where in the brain the toxoplasma lesions form.

Patients who have a positive toxoplasma antibody and a CD4 count less than 100 cells/μL should also receive prophylactic antibiotics to prevent reactivation of this infection. This can be accomplished with Bactrim, the same drug used for PCP prophylaxis. However, if the patient is allergic to Bactrim (a problem that is not uncommon in HIV patients), then a different set of medications needs to be used for both PCP and toxoplasmosis prophylaxis.

Cryptococcus

Cryptococcus is a type of fungus that also is found commonly in the environment. It has been associated with pigeons or other bird droppings. In someone with a depressed level of immunity, cryptococcus can cause several problems, most notably a meningitis—or inflammation of the lining of the brain. This form of meningitis can have a slower onset than meningitis caused by bacteria, which typically have a sudden and dangerously rapid onset and progression. However, left untreated, cryptococcus meningitis is fatal.

Patients with cryptococcal meningitis often complain of headache. They also often develop a stiff neck and a condition called photophobia—or pain when bright light is shined in the eyes. They may develop nausea and vomiting. One of the most dangerous complications of cryptococcal infection is an elevation of the pressure within the head, a problem that can lead to blindness or herniation of the brain out of the skull into the spinal cord. Some patients require repeated spinal taps to remove cerebrospinal fluid (CSF) and thereby decrease the intracranial pressure.

There are no primary prophylactic medications that are used to prevent cryptococcal infection, but if this opportunistic infection occurs, patients are treated aggressively and then remain on a secondary prophylactic medicine called fluconazole to avoid the cryptococcal infection from recurring. This is generally continued until the patient has a rise in their CD4 count out of the more dangerous category, into a level that is sustained above 200 cells/μL for several months.

Infections that can be seen in immunologically "normal" hosts, like tuberculosis, reactivation of varicella zoster virus (the virus that causes chicken pox and then reactivates to cause shingles, a painful rash typically on one side of the body), or bacterial pneumonias, are also more common in HIV-infected persons. Patients may develop thrush, an infection due to a fungus called candida in the mouth, or in the throat. Finally, advanced HIV disease may also be accompanied

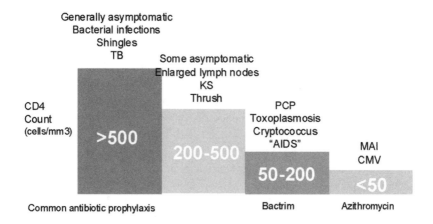

Figure 6.3 Common opportunistic infections and clinical findings by CD4 count. KS = Kaposi's sarcoma. TB = tuberculosis. PCP = pnuemocystis pneumonia. MAI = mycobacterium avium intracellulare. CMV = cytomegalovirus.

by non-infectious problems like weight loss, fatigue, and loss of appetite. Severe weight loss in advanced HIV has been called wasting syndrome. This is what became known as slim disease in some parts of the world like Africa (as we discussed in chapter 3), where this symptom has been severe in untreated persons.

Persons with advanced HIV disease are also at increased risk for developing certain cancers, including cervical or anorectal cancer due to human papillomavirus, Kaposi's sarcoma due to human herpes virus-8, and lymphoma, some forms of which are associated with Ebstein Barr virus. Some other cancers also appear to be more frequent in HIV-infected persons (including lung cancer and Hodgkins lymphoma). Researchers have suggested that this may be due to altered immunologic surveillance for precancerous or cancerous cells—a function which you'll recall is usually handled by T lymphocytes.

Cytomegalovirus

Cytomegalovirus (CMV) is also a reactivation infection, seen most commonly in patients with severe AIDS and a CD4 count below 50 cells/μL. CMV can affect many parts of the body and cause fever, sweats, weight loss, bloody diarrhea, pancreatitis, and neurologic problems including encephalitis or blindness. CMV reactivation in the eye—called CNS retinitis—used to be a fairly common opportunistic infection. But now, with effective antiretroviral therapy, most patients can be prevented from having a CD4 decline to that very low level and can therefore avoid developing CMV retinitis. HIV-positive persons with low CD4 counts should have regular eye exams to guard against this disease and its dangerous consequences. There is no routinely used primary prophylactic medication for this condition. People who develop CMV retinitis are treated with a medicine called gancyclovir that is used both systemically (intravenously or later by pill) as well as intraocularly. This means the medicine is also delivered—by implant—directly into the eye.

These are examples of some of the classic opportunistic infections. Each has its own treatment, and many have their own prophylactic medications to avoid infection. However, the most important way to avoid opportunistic infections is to start and maintain antiretroviral medications against HIV. Treatment of HIV helps to raise the CD4 count and prevent the risk of opportunistic infections in the first place. It is far and away the most important intervention to improve survival in HIV-positive persons with waning CD4 counts.

NONOPPORTUNISTIC COMPLICATIONS OF HIV

Finally, because HIV can spread to every part of the body, complications due to HIV itself can develop over time. HIV can affect the heart, lungs, brain, kidneys, adrenal glands, nerves, and essentially every organ system in the body. HIV can make the heart big, or dilated, and result in ineffective pumping of blood throughout the body. It can cause nodules to form in the lungs (a condition called lymphocytic interstitial pneumonitis, more commonly seen in HIV-infected children), or cause a high pressure in the blood vessels of the lungs (a condition called pulmonary hypertension). HIV has also been associated with early dementia, kidney failure, and inadequate functioning of the adrenal glands. It has been associated with several neurologic conditions, including peripheral neuropathy, which can result in numbness, tingling, pain, or a loss of sensation of the hands and feet.

COINFECTIONS

Special medical consideration is required when HIV coexists with other infections. Here we will examine three examples: (1) HIV and hepatitis (hepatitis B or hepatitis C, the forms that can cause chronic liver infection), (2) HIV and tuberculosis, and (3) HIV and syphilis. In these situations, the presence of HIV may alter the course of the other infection.

HIV and Hepatitis

Coinfection with HIV and hepatitis B or C is a serious problem worldwide. In the United States, about one-third of HIV-infected persons also have hepatitis. Hepatitis B and C is of particular concern because these infections can persist in a chronic state and lead to cirrhosis (a form of liver failure) and/or liver cancer over time. Persons with HIV coinfection are at higher risk for developing the complications of chronic hepatitis infection. They require closer surveillance of liver function and early consideration of treatment of their hepatitis infection. Some of the medicines used to treat HIV are also active against hepatitis B, so the doctor needs to make careful choices about which medicines to use (and in what combination), how to monitor the response of both viruses to the therapy, and when to worry about the development of possible resistance to the medications in both viruses. Guidelines recommend considering treatment implications for both hepatitis B and HIV at the same time in patients who have both infections.

HIV and Tuberculosis

Tuberculosis and HIV coinfection is also a leading problem worldwide. The course of tuberculosis (TB) may be altered by HIV infection. While TB typically presents in the lungs, patients with HIV more commonly have TB in other locations, such as the lymph nodes, the lining of the lungs, the heart, the brain, or disseminated infection throughout the body. TB can also be more difficult to diagnose in HIV-infected persons, because the presence of this coinfection can make the most commonly used test for TB (the purified protein derivative test) falsely negative, since patients lack a strong enough immune system to mount a positive response to the test. TB is also harder to detect on spectrum testing of individuals who are co-infected with HIV. Finally, some of the medications used to treat HIV can have important interactions with the medicines used to treat TB, so the former medications may need to be adjusted and the patient must be monitored closely for signs of medication toxicity, particularly affecting the liver. Because of these important interactions, anyone who is diagnosed with TB should be tested for HIV and vice versa.

HIV and Syphilis

HIV and syphilis requires particular consideration because of its public health implications. Recall from chapter 4 that the presence of ulcerative sexually transmitted diseases (like syphilis) can increase the risk of HIV transmission. Because sexually transmitted diseases can "travel in packs," the presence of one should herald concern and screening for others. This is particularly important because rates of syphilis are on the rise in some communities after many years of decreased transmission. This has become a particular concern in the men-who-have-sex-with-men community. Until the year 2000, syphilis was declining. But now, the CDC reports concerning trends, particularly in MSM groups in several U.S. cities.

Although controversial, some experts believe that coinfection with HIV and syphilis can alter the course of syphilis. HIV-positive persons with syphilis may have a higher rate of relapse, a slower decline after treatment in their laboratory tests for syphilis (with a test called the RPR, or rapid plasma reagin), and possibly more frequent involvement of the central nervous system. The finding of syphilis should also prompt an HIV test, and vice versa.

The diagnosis of a sexually transmitted disease implies exposure to bodily fluids, which increases the risk of HIV transmission, even if there is no genital ulcer disease. It also affords the opportunity for doctors to counsel and educate patients about how to avoid such risks in the future.

SUMMARY

HIV causes a spectrum of illness, starting with the acute retroviral syndrome during acute infection, then a period of relative quiescence, followed by a gradual decline in CD4 counts and the onset of opportunistic infections and complications from untreated HIV itself. All in all, advanced AIDS can affect nearly every part of the body, often with fatal complications if left untreated. As the CD4 count falls, several prophylactic medications should be used to avoid some of the more common opportunistic infections. But the most important intervention is to start effective therapy against HIV and try to raise the CD4 count back into a safer range. HIV can also interact with other infections that coexist in the body at the same time, and careful consideration of possible coinfections is important to ensure adequate treatment of both conditions.

7

Diagnosis and Treatment

Sigall K. Bell, MD

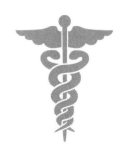

This chapter discusses HIV testing, medications, special health considerations, and potential complications of treatment. We will address the following questions:

- How is HIV diagnosed?
- Who is at risk for HIV infection? Who should get tested?
- What are commonly used medications for HIV and how do they work?
- What are some common side effects of medications?
- How does the virus become resistant to medications? What are the health implications of this problem?
- What effects did the introduction of HIV treatment have on the HIV epidemic?
- What are common complications of HIV medications?
- What is the life expectancy for individuals on HIV treatment?
- What are some other important health issues for people living with HIV (including vaccines, pets, and travel)?

HOW IS HIV DIAGNOSED?

The diagnosis of HIV is made by demonstrating antibodies to this virus in the blood. This is done by a simple blood test. As you recall from earlier chapters, the test is done in two parts, a highly sensitive ELISA followed by a highly specific western blot. A highly sensitive test means that it has few false negatives. In other words, if someone has HIV, the test is unlikely to be negative. A highly specific test means that it has few false positives. In other words, if the test is positive, the patient truly has HIV. The ELISA and western blot tests utilize two different techniques to identify HIV antibodies in the patient's blood. If the ELISA is positive, then a western blot is sent to confirm the ELISA results.

Sometimes a positive ELISA is followed by a negative western blot. This can mean one of the following things: (1) the ELISA was a false positive, (2) the person has very early-stage HIV infection and the body has not yet had enough time to make a full antibody response (making the western blot appear negative), or (3) the person has a different kind of HIV infection (i.e., HIV-2) that is not picked up by the routine western blot. In these cases, the first step is to repeat the western blot several weeks later. If the patient had an exposure that is epidemiologically linked with HIV-2 (which you will recall is predominantly found in West Africa), then a different test, the HIV-2 western blot should be done. If the HIV-1 or HIV-2 western blot is still negative by 6 to 12 months, then the person does not have HIV and the test is considered a false positive result.

Thought Box

If you were designing an HIV test, would you make it highly sensitive or highly specific? What are the advantages and disadvantages of each, particularly as it pertains to a test for HIV? What is the rationale for combining a highly sensitive and highly specific test?

WHO SHOULD BE TESTED FOR HIV?

The traditional thinking about HIV testing was that anyone who fell into a high-risk category (Table 7.1) should be tested. This includes people who have multiple sex partners, men who have sex with men, IV drug users, children of HIV+ mothers, people who develop "AIDS defining" illnesses, or the sexual partners of high-risk persons. People who develop certain concerning clinical signs and symptoms were also considered high priority for testing (Table 7.1). However, in September 2006, the Centers for Disease Control (CDC) announced that HIV testing should be universal, recommending that HIV testing should become a routine part of medical care. The CDC estimates that one-quarter of the U.S. HIV epidemic is undiagnosed. Universal screening aims to find these previously

Table 7.1 Traditional Indications for HIV Antibody Testing

Traditional Historical Risk-Factor Based Indications for HIV Testing

---

- Men who have sex with men
- Persons with multiple sexual partners
- Current or past injection drug users
- Recipients of blood products between 1978 and 1985
- Persons with current or past sexually transmitted diseases
- Commercial sex workers and their contacts
- Pregnant women and women of child-bearing age
- Children born to HIV-infected mothers
- Sexual partners of those at risk for HIV infection
- Donors of blood products, semen, or organs
- Persons who consider themselves at risk or request testing

Traditional Clinical Indications for HIV Testing

- Tuberculosis
- Syphilis
- Recurrent shingles
- Chronic constitutional symptoms like fever, weight loss, night sweats
- Chronic generalized adenopathy
- Chronic diarrhea or wasting
- Encephalopathy
- Thrombocytopenia
- Unexplained thrush or chronic/recurrent vaginal candida infections
- HIV-associated opportunistic diseases (i.e., PCP, MAI, CMV, Toxoplasmosis, etc.)

---

undiagnosed cases in order to connect those individuals that have HIV but don't know it with appropriate health care. It also aims to prevent further spread of HIV—"unknowingly"—from those individuals who do not know they have HIV to other people.

MEDICATIONS FOR HIV

When should HIV infection be treated? The threshold for starting HIV medications has shifted over the years ranging from recommendations to start treatment when the CD4 count is less than or equal to 200, to more recent recommendations to start when the CD4 count falls below 500. Some experts even suggest starting when the CD4 is above 500. Experts making such recommendations try to balance the toxicity and long-term complications of HIV medications against potential harm of untreated infection, even when CD4 counts are relatively high. With improved medications and more recent insights into the potential problems of unchecked HIV replication and its effects on the body, the pendulum is swinging toward earlier treatment.

Doctors, in discussion with their patients, can help guide the right time to start medications. In addition to the CD4 threshold, several other factors guide the timing of initiation of medications in the United States. For example, it is important that the patient is ready, willing, and able to start and stay on medications since sporadic use can be harmful, by generating resistance to those medications, as we will soon discuss. Mental illness, drug use, homelessness, or other such issues may present significant challenges. Pregnant women should be started on ART irrespective of the CD4 count, to help prevent transmission to the fetus. The same is true for persons with Hepatitis B infection that requires treatment (since the drugs used to treat hepatitis B may also be active against HIV) and for persons with kidney disease due to HIV infection. Anyone with a prior AIDS-defining illness should also be on treatment. Persons with active symptoms due to HIV disease, especially individuals with acute HIV infection or recent acquisition of infection (i.e., in the last 6 months) should also be considered for treatment. These recommendations are frequently updated—if you are interested in learning more, check out: http://www.aidsinfo.nih.gov/guidelines/.

Medications used to treat HIV are called antiretrovirals. They have this name because they target the HIV virus, which you recall from chapter 1 is a retrovirus. There are over 25 antiretroviral medications to treat HIV, belonging to several different classes. The drugs were developed to block different stages of HIV replication and to act at several of the steps in the viral replication cycle that we reviewed in chapter 2. We will review each of these classes briefly and you can see how they work by looking at where they act in the HIV life cycle (see Figure 2.2). The goal of HIV treatment is to control the virus—stopping it from making copies of itself and therefore stopping it from harming the body. However, there is currently no cure for HIV.

Remember that when HIV enters a human cell it can do one of two things: either it begins to replicate, releasing many more copies of virus into the body, or it can integrate itself into the host cell DNA and remain dormant indefinitely as pro-DNA. The latter situation is a good news/bad news scenario. Because the HIV is dormant, it is not replicating and releasing more virus into the body. However, because it is not replicating or "showing itself" to the body, it is very hard for the body to find it and attack it. As a result, it is able to hide and survive. The ability of HIV to integrate into the human cell DNA and remain undetected by the body is one reason that there currently is no cure. All it takes is for one cell containing the integrated HIV pro-DNA to activate and start replicating for the infection to become widespread again.

Nucleoside Reverse Transcriptase Inhibitors

The first class of drugs developed to fight HIV was the NRTIs: nucleoside reverse transcriptase inhibitors. These drugs look like the base pair building blocks of HIV, but they are "chain terminators." They integrate into the growing chain of the HIV genome when it is replicating, but, rather than allow the chain to continue to grow, they terminate replication. This means that the virus can no longer make a functional copy of itself. There are several drugs in this class. Perhaps the most famous one is AZT (also called ZDV or zidovudine), because it was the first drug that was ever found to be effective against HIV. As more drugs were developed, AZT was used in combination with other medications. Even though it was discovered many years ago, today it is still an important part of HIV treatment regimens for some patients. You will recall that it also has a key role in prevention of mother-to-child transmission. AZT has been a key medicine since it was first discovered. However, it can cause several common side effects, including headache, nausea, vomiting, and dizziness. It can also lower the red blood cell count, causing anemia, or a particular subset of white blood cells called neutrophils, causing neutropenia.

Non-Nucleoside Reverse Transcriptase Inhibitors

Another class of drugs is the NNRTIs: non-nucleoside reverse transcriptase inhibitors. These drugs also interfere with the chain elongation of the HIV genome, but they do it in a slightly different way. These medications are highly effective when used in combination with other HIV medications, but the virus is able to quickly develop resistance to this class of medication if they are used alone or if patients do not take their medications regularly. We will talk more about resistance later in this chapter. We already talked about one drug in this class of medications: nevirapine. It is another important medicine used for the prevention of mother-to-child transmission.

The NNRTIs as a class are generally well-tolerated, which means they may not have a lot of side effects. However, one member of this class—efaverinz—has a peculiar side effect: it causes bizarre, vivid dreams. In addition to potentially causing dizziness, especially when it is first started, the medicine can lead to these unusual dreams. Sometimes they come in the form of nightmares, and the patient and doctor will then work together to see if there is a different medicine that can be substituted. Since efaverinz is such a potent, effective drug, and only needs to be taken once a day, many patients are willing to try this medicine and work through the bizarre dreams. Usually if a patient can stay on the medicine for the first few weeks, the effect goes away or is at least lessened. Efaverinz is also included as part of a combination pill with two other medicines packaged into one single pill. This means the patient can take three medicines in one pill once a day—dramatic progress in HIV treatment.

Protease Inhibitors

The PIs—protease inhibitors—are a third class of HIV medications. These medications inhibit the enzyme protease, which is needed by the virus to package up all of the viral particles after they have been replicated into new discrete HIV viruses. Protease is a key enzyme for organizing new viruses so that they can then leave the infected cell and enter a new one to begin the replication process all over again. The protease inhibitors are powerful, effective medicines, but they can have many side effects. Diarrhea is common. Also, the protease inhibitors can have detrimental effects like raising cholesterol levels—a condition that can lead to heart disease, and causing poor blood sugar control, which can result in diabetes.

Entry Inhibitors

The entry inhibitors were designed to try to prevent HIV from entering the cell. Some people consider fusion inhibitors and CCR5 inhibitors separately, each as their own class, but for our purposes we will include both fusion inhibitors and CCR5 inhibitors together, since they both effectively help to prevent entry of the virus into the cell. CCR5 inhibitors block the binding step of HIV with the human cell CCR5 coreceptor, a step necessary for HIV to enter the cell. Remember that in chapter 2 we discussed the HIV coreceptors CCR5 and CXCR4. As you can imagine, the CCR5 inhibitors are only active against those strains of HIV that use the CCR5 receptor. Before starting this medicine, a special test called a tropism assay is used to determine which coreceptor HIV is using in a given patient, to make sure he or she is an appropriate candidate for this medicine. Fusion inhibitors prevent the HIV envelope from fusing with the human cell. The most commonly used fusion inhibitor is a drug called T-20. It has a limited role in treatment because it is mostly called upon in so-called salvage regimens, when other front-line medicines are no longer working (mostly because of the problem of viral resistance). This medication needs to be injected subcutaneously twice a day, so it incurs a significant burden on quality of life for patients using this drug as part of their regimen.

Integrase Inhibitors

One of the newest classes of medications is the integrase inhibitors. These medications target the integrase enzyme and prevent HIV from integrating into the human cell DNA in the nucleus of the cell. By stopping this crucial step, the virus cannot replicate itself, since it relies on the host cell machinery to make copies of itself. The integrase inhibitors are generally well-tolerated, without many side effects, although they can cause an elevation in liver function tests.

HIV MEDICATION COMBINATIONS

AZT was approved for use in 1990. Initially it was used alone. As other HIV medications became available, doctors prescribed them in combination—to increase their effectiveness against the virus. At first two drugs were used at a time, and then three drugs were used together. As new classes of drugs became available, particularly the NNRTIs and the PIs, researchers found that using a combination of two NRTIs and one PI or NNRTI could significantly enhance survival of HIV-infected persons. As patients started to take these HIV medication "cocktails," as they were called at the time, a remarkable thing happened: The death rate from AIDS showed a sudden and steep decline (see Figure 7.1). The combination of three medications was coined HAART, standing for highly active antiretroviral therapy. HIV-positive patients started living longer and regaining enough health to go back to work, have children, and live essentially normal lives. People who were on the verge of "settling their affairs" and saying goodbye to their friends and family just before 1995–1996 when the "cocktail" became available suddenly had a new lease on life.

The other big advance in HIV medication is the development of drugs that are easier to take. In the early part of the epidemic, people had to take handfuls of pills several times a day. Many set alarm clocks throughout the day and night to remember to take all their pills. They had many bad side effects including severe nausea, vomiting, diarrhea, and problems with lowered blood counts due to effects of the drugs. But scientists worked hard to develop new medications that would be more effective and less toxic to patients. They also manufactured formulations of combination pills—medications that had two or even three HIV drugs all in one pill. This decreased the so-called pill burden significantly, making it easier for patients to take all their medications. They also worked on making

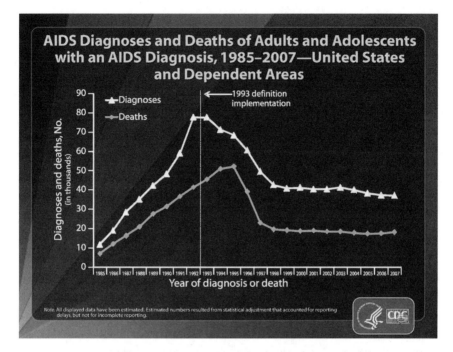

Figure 7.1 Estimated AIDS diagnosis and deaths of adults and adolescents from 1985–2007 in the United States. (Centers for Disease Control)

medications that could last longer, so they could be taken just once a day, rather than the four-times-a-day requirement of the earliest medications.

The pace and ingenuity of HIV medication development was remarkable. HIV activist groups knew that new medications were necessary to save lives, at a time when the death toll from HIV was dramatic. They pushed hard to drive progress and to help patients gain access to new drugs as soon as possible. Over a period of less than 20 years after the discovery of AZT, about 30 drugs and combination pills were developed, tested, and approved—an extraordinary part of the HIV story. The most dramatic advancement was the development of a single combination pill that contains three HIV medications and can be taken once a day, as mentioned in the section on NNRTIs. Compared to the early 1990s, when HIV-positive patients had to take handfuls of medications several times a day, and tolerate many difficult side effects, today's HIV-positive patients can potentially take a regimen as simple as one pill a day, with relatively fewer side effects.

HIV MUTATIONS AND RESISTANCE

Using three drugs at once to fight HIV proved to be a critical step—not only because it increased the effectiveness of the treatment, but also because it helped to decrease the rapid acquisition of resistance to the medications. What do we mean by resistance? Resistance is a term used to describe what happens when the virus changes itself so that certain medications no longer work. How does it do this?

Remember that the HIV medications work at several different steps in the viral life cycle. Remember also that HIV comes "packaged" with its own reverse transcriptase (RT), the enzyme that helps HIV replicate by using the host cell machinery to make more copies of itself. In earlier chapters we discussed the fact that RT is "error-prone"; in other words, it makes lots of mistakes, about one mistake for every 2,000 base pairs that it replicates. Since the HIV genome has 9,000 base pairs, and HIV can replicate itself billions of times per day, this introduces lots of opportunities for changes in the virus's genetic blueprint. Some of these mistakes, or mutations, harm the virus and prevent it from making normal copies of itself. But some of the mistakes turn out to be good for the virus. Imagine for example if RT makes a mistake at a critical base pair, one that results in a change in shape at the site where a medication usually binds. Now that medication can no longer bind, or it doesn't bind well. The virus is now less susceptible to that medication: it has developed some resistance.

While spontaneous mutations such as the one just described do occur occasionally, the most common and problematic way that resistance develops is when a patient who is on HIV medications does not take them regularly. This results in subtherapeutic—or below effective—levels of medicine. Missing doses allows the virus to take advantage of lulls in medication when the drug levels are not high enough to suppress the virus and to develop mutations against those drugs. Those viruses that adapt to survive through the "selective pressure" of the low level of medicine have an advantage and therefore go on to produce more viruses just like themselves—all with new resistance to the medicine that wasn't present in high enough doses to kill the virus. The best way to avoid this problem is to reinforce how important regular adherence to medications is for maintaining HIV control. Doctors will often review how patients are doing with their medications, and if they missed any doses, for exactly this reason.

The third way that resistance develops is if patients take medications that are only partially active against their strain of virus. Let's imagine that a patient already has some resistance mutations, and the patient is taking a medication regimen that is therefore not completely effective. In this situation, the virus may only be effectively "seeing" one or two medications. As the virus replicates against the selective pressure of partially active medications, it can take advantage of mutations that help it to escape from these medications. There are not three fully active drugs to help prevent the emergence of resistance. In other words, the only partially active drugs can make it easier for resistance to emerge to the fully active drug(s).

For these reasons, it is extremely important that doctors monitor the level of virus very carefully and respond to any signs of inactive or partially active drugs right away. It is also crucial that patients understand the importance of taking their medications regularly and that the health-care team works closely with patients to prevent them from missing doses.

Resistance is a very serious problem in HIV care. When resistance to drugs develops, the viral load climbs higher because the virus is able to replicate. The goal of HIV treatment is to drive the level of virus to undetectable levels. This means that when the viral load blood test is done to detect the virus in the bloodstream, the level of virus will be below the limit of the test's detection. As you recall, since there currently isn't a cure for HIV, this does not mean that there is no HIV present. It simply means that the level of virus in the blood is so low, the test can not pick it up. When the viral load becomes detectable, doctors will do resistance testing to see which medications the virus has become resistant to and whether they need to find different medications that the patient can take in order to control the virus. Depending on how much resistance there is, this can be difficult, especially since some of the mutations that the virus develops can make it resistant to several different medications, or even to a whole class of medications. Even though there are now many more HIV medication options available than there used to be, a patient can run out of drug choices relatively quickly.

RT can make mistakes, or genetic mutations, in the viral genome that allows it to survive better in other ways too. In addition to escaping from medications, the virus can also escape from the human immune system. Although most human immune systems cannot control HIV in the long term without the help of medications, the immune system does mount a substantial fight against HIV to contribute to viral control. As RT makes mistakes, it can change the shape of a key viral particle that the immune system typically "sees" and attacks (such as key protein "flags" on its surface, making it no longer "recognizable" to the immune system. The virus has masked itself and hides from the immune system. It can also develop a mutation at a key site on the virus where the immune systems fighter cells usually bind to the virus in order to destroy it. If they can't bind with the virus, they have a harder time destroying the virus or the cell it has infected.

MEDICATION SIDE EFFECTS

As we discussed earlier, the side effects from HIV medications have become much less severe than they used to be, but still, many significant potential reactions to the drugs exist. We can think about side effects to HIV medications in two categories: those that occur relatively early and those that occur with long-term use.

Early HIV Medication Reactions

Many of the HIV medications still can cause stomach and bowel problems, like nausea, vomiting, or diarrhea. Often, if a person can tolerate these symptoms for the first couple of weeks after starting a new HIV medication, the symptoms get better. Other early reactions can include rash, headache, dizziness, bizarre dreams, kidney or liver problems, or fatigue. However, for the most part, patients today do relatively well with HIV medications, especially once their body adjusts to the new medicines.

One other potential HIV medication reaction is called the Immune Reconstitution Inflammatory Syndrome (IRIS). This complication can occur shortly after starting HIV medications, usually within weeks to months. Because the medications help combat HIV and strengthen the immune system, the patient may suddenly have a paradoxical flare in pre-existing opportunistic infections or other conditions that were previously more quiescent, owing to the person's relative lack of immune fighter cells. Armed with more and stronger CD4 T cells as a result of treatment, the patient may develop new or exacerbated symptoms. While IRIS has been reported with many opportunistic infections (OIs), as well as non-OI conditions like thyroid disease, it can classically cause flares in PCP, CMV, TB, Cryptococcus, and MAI (OIs we discussed in chapter 6). Since the symptoms are caused by the body's new capacity to mount an inflammatory reaction to these infections, they can often be controlled with anti-inflammatory medications.

Long-Term Complications of HIV Medication Use

There are several important potential long-term complications of HIV medication use. These can affect nearly any organ in the human body. Let's talk about a few of the particularly notable ones.

Diabetes

Diabetes is a condition that develops when the body cannot control the level of sugar in the blood appropriately. As a result, the blood sugar can get too high and cause damage to the eyes, heart, kidneys, nervous system, and blood vessels. Some of the HIV medications, especially the PI group, can predispose a patient to develop diabetes. Patients on HIV medications should therefore have their blood sugar monitored closely to prevent this complication.

Lactic Acidosis

An uncommon, but dangerous complication of HAART is a condition called lactic acidosis. HIV medications target HIV itself and therefore do not generally impair the normal replication of human DNA. Remember that several of the HIV medications target the HIV reverse transcriptase enzyme that is used to replicate HIV RNA. While HIV medications do not affect human DNA polymerase enzymes, they can affect an enzyme called polymerase gamma, which is found in mitochondria. Mitochondria are the energy-generating factories located in human cells. While most of the human cell DNA is located in the cell nucleus, mitochondria have their own DNA. These mitochondria may be damaged by HIV medications resulting in malfunction. When mitochondria are damaged, too much lactate—a natural byproduct of metabolism of glucose—can build up and cause a potentially life-threatening condition. Symptoms of mitochondrial toxicity or lactic acidosis can be vague, including nausea or vomiting, shortness of breath, abdominal pain, or dizziness. Some researchers believe that conditions such as lipodystrophy and hepatic steatosis (also called "fatty liver"), are also linked to mitochondrial toxicity.

Osteopenia

Osteopenia refers to loss of bone. In severe forms, osteopenia can progress to osteoporosis, the problem that some elderly or ill people encounter when they lose bone density, predisposing them to fractures—especially at the spine or hip. Several HIV medications can cause osteopenia, although this condition is less common than some of the other complications, like high cholesterol.

Hypercholesterolemia

Several of the HIV medications from many different classes (but especially the PIs and some NRTIs) can cause abnormalities in lipid metabolism. This can result in very high levels of cholesterol and/or triglycerides. As you may know, high levels of these fats in the blood can predispose a person to developing serious medical problems such as a heart attack, pancreatitis, or stroke. People taking HIV medications should have their cholesterol and other lipid levels monitored closely by simple blood tests at least once a year in order to detect any problematic changes early and take the necessary steps to bring the levels back down.

Neuropathy

A few of the older NRTIs were capable of causing damage to the nerves, a condition called neuropathy. The nerves first affected are the longest ones, the ones reaching the toes or the fingers, a distribution called "stocking-glove" and characteristic of peripheral neuropathy. Patients who develop peripheral neuropathy will complain of pain or numbness and tingling affecting their fingers and/or toes. It is important to detect this early because some neuropathy is reversible if the medications are stopped quickly, but the symptoms may persist if the drug is continued long-term.

Lipodystrophy

Long-term exposure to HIV medications can lead to a condition called lipodystrophy. Generally speaking, lipodystrophy has been used as a catch phrase for to two problems: too much fat deposition in some places and too little in others (although the latter condition has its own term: lipoatrophy). In some patients who take HIV medications for a long time the distribution of body fat is rearranged so that there is more in central locations, like around the belly or upper back, but less in peripheral locations like the arms and legs. Patients can develop a "buffalo hump," which is an enlargement of the dorsocervical fat pad, located at the back of the neck and top of the back. This complication is much less common today with the more advanced HIV medications than it was earlier in the epidemic when the older PI drugs were found to cause this problem. However, many patients do still notice increased fat around the midsection of their bodies or thinning of the arms and legs, such that the veins and muscles are particularly prominent. Some also notice a thinning of the face, particularly around the cheeks and nose.

Lipodystrophy can be prevented by doctors who monitor closely for body changes that they see or that the patient notices. When these occur, they will often consider changing medications to try to find a regimen that is more "friendly" to the fat distribution pattern. This may be different for each person, although there are certain medications that have a higher risk of causing lipodystrophy. You might be thinking, if this is the case, why not use those lower-risk medications for everyone? The problem is that each medication comes with its own set of potential long-term problems. One that is better for lipodystrophy might be worse for the kidney or the heart, for example. Doctors have to choose the medicine that makes the most sense for each individual patient, depending on their own particular set of medical issues.

Heart Disease

Both HIV itself and the medications used to treat it can accelerate heart disease. This means that patients are at risk for developing insufficient blood flow to the heart or even a heart attack at a younger age than is typically seen. This serious complication can be avoided by focusing on reducing other cardiovascular risk factors. The most important risk factors that can be modified by healthy behaviors include avoiding smoking, high blood pressure (which can be decreased by keeping weight at a healthy range for example), high cholesterol, and diabetes. Several of these risk factors for heart disease can be decreased with a healthy low-fat diet and regular aerobic exercise. Sometimes doctors will also recommend changing some HIV medications if they are contributing to worsening some of these risk factors, such as high cholesterol or diabetes.

COMPLICATIONS OF HIV DISEASE

HIV can affect nearly every organ in the body. In addition to causing a weakening of the immune system, left untreated it can cause many problems due to direct effects of the virus, or due to the general "inflammatory state" and "revved up" immune system it creates. Such chronic inflammation can harm the body. Some long term complications of HIV include kidney failure and a decline in brain function (dementia), among other problems. It can enter the bone marrow and cause a decrease in the blood cells that are formed there, as well as bone loss. In addition to increasing the risk of a heart attack, HIV can also cause a decrease in the function of the heart, making it unable to squeeze blood through its chambers and out to the circulation as well as it normally does. This condition is called cardiomyopathy. The most common form of cardiomyopathy caused by HIV is called dilated cardiomyopathy, in which the chambers of the heart become enlarged like a stretched-out balloon. HIV also increases the risks of developing several kinds of cancer, including cancer of the lung, cervix, anus, brain, lymph nodes, and others. For all these reasons, a person who has HIV requires close follow-up with their doctor. HIV medications have dramatically changed both the life expectancy and the quality of life of persons with HIV by preventing both degradation of the immune system as well as some of the complications of HIV affecting other parts of the body.

LIFE EXPECTANCY AND IMPORTANT HEALTH ISSUES

Although HIV was once a fatal diagnosis, it has now become what we call a chronic illness in countries with access to effective antiretroviral therapy, meaning people can live with HIV for many years—just like other long-term conditions such as high blood pressure or diabetes—as long as they take their medications regularly and visit doctors routinely to check in on their health. Because people with HIV are living longer and longer, it also becomes increasingly important to pay attention to screening for the usual health problems that can develop with older age, like heart disease, cancer, and osteoporosis, especially since HIV can increase the risk for some of these conditions.

Vaccines

Protective vaccines are an important way to keep people healthy. People with HIV should get a flu (or influenza) vaccine each year and should also receive a pneumonia vaccine. Vaccines against hepatitis B and, in some cases, hepatitis A, are also recommended. They should get tetanus vaccine boosters every 10 years, just like all other adults.

Vaccines come in two forms: inactivated and live attenuated. Inactivated vaccines do not have any live components. They use protein or polysaccharide particles to help the vaccine recipients mount an immune response to the target infection, like influenza, pneumococcus (a bacteria that causes pneumonia), hepatitis A and B, and so on. The live attenuated vaccines work a little differently. These vaccines actually contain a live virus or bacterium that has been attenuated, or weakened, so that it does not cause harm to a normal human host. Because persons with HIV may have a weakened immune system, they have to be very careful with live vaccines, because even though the virus or bacteria are attenuated, they can still cause disease in persons with decreased immunity. These vaccines, which include varicella, zoster, measles-mumps-rubella, inhaled influenza vaccine, and yellow fever, should generally be avoided unless carefully reviewed by a doctor. Some people with HIV can receive some of these vaccines, especially if their CD4 count—the laboratory marker of the strength of the immune system—is high. If a household member of someone with HIV is receiving a live vaccine, extra precautions may also be required to prevent exposure to the HIV-positive person. The presence of an immunocompromised household member should be discussed with the doctor at the time of the planned vaccine to ensure that it is safe to proceed.

An increased life expectancy has given persons with HIV an opportunity to enjoy many experiences, including travel, pets, and having a family. The best way to ensure a safe experience in each of these areas is to plan ahead of time with the help of a doctor.

Travel

Today, many HIV-positive patients can travel safely, even to remote destinations or to areas where additional health risks like malaria or typhoid fever are endemic. Like HIV-negative persons, these patients should meet with a doctor specializing in travel medicine to receive the necessary and permissible vaccines and medications to prepare for their trip.

Pets

HIV-positive persons can develop and sustain healthy relationships with pets, but extra precautions are sometimes needed. Exposure to certain animals can increase the risk of particular infections, to which persons with compromised immune systems are even more susceptible. For example, turtles can carry salmonella, kittens can transmit toxoplasmosis, puppies can have cryptosporidium infection, and several birds can put their owner at risk for histoplasmosis or psiticcosis (a type of chlamydia infection that affects the lungs). It's particularly important to have the pet thoroughly checked by a vet, and often helpful to have someone else change the cat litter or clean the bird cage, for example. Careful attention to hand-washing after handling pets and other preventive measures are critical.

Having a Family

As you recall from chapter 5, HIV can be transmitted sexually, and also from mother to fetus. Fortunately, with today's advances, HIV-positive persons who want to have children can do so with greatly reduced risk of transmission between sexual partners or between mother and child. The first key to reducing transmission is achieving an undetectable HIV viral load by having the HIV-positive person take highly active antiretroviral therapy. If the father-to-be is HIV positive, special techniques like sperm washing, followed by intrauterine insemination, can be used to help remove HIV from the semen. If the mother-to-be is HIV positive, intrauterine insemination may also be considered. In cases where the mother is HIV positive, HIV medications are generally recommended in the U.S. throughout pregnancy and delivery, regardless of the mother's CD4 count or other usual criteria used to decide whether to start treatment, in order to decrease risk of transmission to the baby. Some doctors will recommend delivery by Caesarian section to further decrease risk to the baby if the mother's viral load is detectable at a particular threshold at the time of delivery. When all precautions are taken effectively, the risk of transmission to the baby can be decreased to less than 1 percent.

Many doctors and many countries recommend routine HIV testing of all pregnant women. Many clinics have adopted an opt-out program, which means that a mother will be tested very early in prenatal care unless she specifically requests not to be tested. Using opt-out testing, any mother who has HIV can be diagnosed as soon as possible so that she can be treated right away and therefore decrease the risk of the baby becoming HIV-infected. If despite these efforts the mother is first found to be HIV positive at the time of delivery, medications can be used during delivery (given to the mother and then to the newborn child) to try to decrease transmission. The delivery of these medications stems from studies that have shown success in decreasing transmission and are now part of maternal to child transmission (MTCT) reduction programs worldwide, as discussed in chapter 9.

SUMMARY

We have come a very long way in HIV diagnosis and treatment. Antiretroviral medications today are much more advanced, but still some significant side effects and long-term complications can occur. Building a strong relationship with a doctor specialized in HIV disease is important for HIV-positive patients so that he or she can carefully monitor and review any changes in HIV control and make critical changes in medicines early enough to prevent the emergence of viral resistance. For their part, patients can also prevent resistance by taking their medications regularly and avoiding missed doses. Because of effective treatment for HIV, patients today can have a long life expectancy and enjoy many life activities, including having a family, pets, and travel, as long as they do so with the close guidance of their doctors.

8

Cultural Impact of HIV

Courtney L. McMickens, MD, MPH

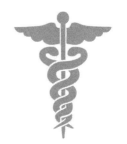

This chapter explores the impact of HIV on society. In it we will probe the following questions:

- What were the early reactions to HIV?
- What lends to social stigma of disease, and what was it like in the case of HIV?
- Who was Ryan White, and how did his story affect the HIV epidemic?
- How did Magic Johnson affect the way we think about HIV?
- What are some global problems related to HIV?
  - Population effects
  - Economic effects
  - The orphan crisis
  - Barriers to treatment

EARLY REACTIONS TO HIV

In order to explore in depth the early reactions to HIV, let's go back in time (and to chapter 1) to remind ourselves how the first cases of HIV were discovered.

Although it did not yet have a name, cases of what is now known to be HIV/ AIDS were first recognized in the summer of 1981, with localized outbreaks in New York and California of rare opportunistic illnesses that were being diagnosed in young previously healthy males. These conditions included the cancer Kaposi's sarcoma, and pneumocystis pneumonia (PCP). Because the clusters of Kaposi's sarcoma and PCP were primarily among young gay men, it was assumed that this syndrome was a disease of homosexual men and could not be transmitted to heterosexuals and women. The disease was even referred to as the gay-related immune deficiency (GRID) in the early 1980s.

In December 1981, a case of PCP was documented in an injection drug user. Cases were then reported among Haitians and hemophiliacs in 1982. One year after the initial diagnosis of opportunistic conditions occurring in clusters in the United States there were 452 cases in 23 states. At this point, it was clear that the disease was not exclusively a disease of homosexual men, but one that could decrease the ability to fight off other diseases in anyone that was infected. Therefore, the disease was given a new name: acquired immunodeficiency syndrome (AIDS). The source of AIDS remained unknown. There was some speculation that the disease may be sexually transmitted due to its prevalence among homosexual men, but that did not explain everything. When an infant died of AIDS following multiple transfusions, researchers began to suspect that the source may be an infectious agent, such as bacteria or virus, that could be found in blood.

By 1983, AIDS cases had been reported in the United States, Europe, and several African countries. Several cases were also reported in Haiti, which led to unsupported claims that AIDS originated in Haiti and to an informal classification of HIV high-risk groups as the "4-H club"—homosexuals, hemophiliacs, heroin addicts, and Haitians. This fueled discrimination and stigmatization toward these groups. Some Haitian Americans lost their jobs and homes. It also caused Haiti to suffer from a dramatic decrease in tourism. Children with hemophilia were withdrawn from summer camps and forced to leave school because parents refused to send their children to school with a child that might be HIV positive.

The increasing prevalence of AIDS among marginalized and isolated populations caused other more mainstream members of society to feel that they were not at risk. Many assumed that AIDS was not "their" disease. Casting shame and blame on others was a consistent early reaction to AIDS and had deep lasting effects on the populations who were stigmatized. The stigma was so profound that it ultimately resulted in the creation of laws to protect those with HIV against discrimination due to stigma and ignorance about this new disease.

The epidemic would soon touch the lives of individuals all around the world, and it became apparent that this was a disease that could not be ignored. Travel, commerce, and globalization had indeed made the world a small place in the 20th century, and country borders could not put boundaries on the spread of disease. Recognizing the global ramifications of this illness, the Institute for Healthcare Improvement's former President Don Berwick urged everyone to become involved in the fight against AIDS in his article, "We All Have AIDS." He made the argument that it is everyone's responsibility and in everyone's best interest to participate in the fight against AIDS. Blame and lack of awareness were no longer acceptable, he argued.

The discovery of the virus responsible for AIDS in 1983, and a test to detect HIV in the blood in 1985 were landmark achievements. But although these were great advances in the characterization, detection, and prevention of AIDS, there were still several unknowns remaining.

The early years of HIV and AIDS were plagued by fear and ignorance regarding the risk of disease transmission. As the number of AIDS cases increased around the world, anxiety increased among the general public. In spite of announcements form the national Centers of Disease Control (CDC) that HIV could not be spread through casual contact, HIV-positive individuals were evicted from their homes, and banned from several public settings or community activities, such as taking communion wine. Children with HIV were not allowed to attend school.

As the prevalence of AIDS increased among both men and women, it became clear that HIV could spread just as easily via heterosexuals as it had among homosexuals. Over the next several years, researchers concluded that HIV could be transmitted not only via sexual intercourse, but also by sharing needles with infected individuals, and by transfusion of contaminated blood and blood products, including from an infected mother to her child during pregnancy. The idea that HIV could be transmitted as a result of casual contact was eventually dispelled. However, false beliefs have been difficult to eradicate. Public images, such as those of AIDS-conference protestors being arrested by gloved police officers, may have reinforced misconceptions about mechanisms of transmission. In the summer of 2006, a homeless man who claimed to be HIV positive spit in the face of a police officer, and he was later sentenced to 35 years in prison for assault with a "deadly weapon: his saliva." This sentencing, in spite of the overwhelming evidence that there is an extremely low/negligible risk of HIV transmission as a result of this act, sent the public mixed messages about the risks of HIV transmission.

Partially in response to the skewed public perception of this disease and the victimization of HIV-infected individuals, as well as with the goal of limiting the disease's spread, multiple AIDS-related organizations emerged around the world to focus on education. The first annual International Conference on AIDS was held in 1985 and was followed by an international meeting organized by the World Health Organization (WHO) on the AIDS pandemic, to lead a collaborative international effort to fight the devastation due to the disease. Campaigns on HIV prevention rolled out around the world. Condom use or abstinence became key components of preventive messages.

As treatments for HIV became available, how to distribute these expensive medications became the topic of debate. There were disagreements among countries and drug companies regarding the cost and the method by which the drugs should be distributed. Many felt that it was an ethical imperative for drug companies to provide this life-saving medication to poor countries, even at extremely discounted prices, but others resisted. Drug prices were reduced, but the distribution of drugs in developing countries remained substandard.

Dr. Berwick has been a prominent leader and activist. In addition to encouraging ongoing education about HIV and empathy toward those affected by the disease, he urged pharmaceutical companies to lower the prices of antiretroviral drugs for the treatment of HIV in poor countries.

Thought Box

Do you think drug companies have a responsibility to provide free HIV medications to countries that cannot afford them?

SOCIAL STIGMA

Stigma is defined as a mark of shame or discredit. Due to the emergence of AIDS among marginalized populations and the initial ignorance about its mechanism of transmission, stigma has been strongly associated with HIV and AIDS. In the early years, people assumed that those infected with HIV "brought it upon themselves" by being sexually irresponsible or by using illegal drugs. There was often a clear distinction in people's minds between HIV-infected people who acquired the disease through their own behaviors as compared to babies or blood transfusion recipients who were infected through "no fault of their own."

Although hemophiliacs were often viewed as innocent victims, they were still barred from school and were socially isolated because of fear that they would infect others through casual contact. HIV-positive individuals were often denied health insurance, health care, and jobs, and some were even violently attacked. A Florida family with three sons who had contracted HIV from blood transfusions for hemophilia was forced to move from Florida in order to try to get the boys into school. The boys were still denied admission to school. The family also received threats from individuals in their community, and their house was set on fire.

Stigma has also had a significant impact on the transmission of the disease. Due to the social attacks against those with HIV, volunteer testing was avoided by people who thought they may be at risk because they feared public reaction to even the *possibility* of testing positive. As a result, many who were HIV-positive remained unaware of their status and unknowingly spread the virus to others.

Stigma also hindered medical follow-up and drug adherence. You'll recall from chapter 7 that in the past, HIV drug regimens were quite complicated and required taking multiple pills throughout the day. It was difficult to take the medications at school or at work without someone noticing and getting suspicious. Multiple visits to the doctor or hospitalizations were also viewed as a clue to the presence of the illness. Some HIV-positive individuals did not adhere to medical care for fear of social isolation or discrimination. Because HIV medications require strict adherence to avoid the emergence of resistant strains, undertreated or partially treated HIV-positive individuals presented a possible risk of spreading a resistant strain of the virus to others.

As the HIV epidemic evolved, so did the cultural response to the disease. Although HIV-related stigma still exists today in some settings, it has been dramatically decreased. Several public icons and human stories have helped to shape public awareness and transform societal attitudes. A few examples are discussed here.

THE RYAN WHITE STORY

Nightline's Ted Koppel described this teenager as "an extraordinary young man; brave, tolerant and wise beyond his years." Ryan White, diagnosed with AIDS in 1984 at the age of 13, appeared on the show after grasping the world's attention by his fight to attend school. Ryan was infected with HIV as the result of a transfusion of blood products to treat his hemophilia. He was diagnosed after he developed PCP associated with AIDS. He was told he had less than a year to live. Ryan decided that he wanted to spend his remaining time living the life of a normal teenager, which included attending school and having fun with his friends, but he was barred from attending school because of his HIV status.

Ryan was forced to go to court in order to return to school after a nine-month absence. He agreed to use separate restrooms, drinking fountains, and disposable eating utensils and trays to appease teachers, parents, and administrators. Upon his return, Ryan was harassed by his classmates. Some parents withdrew their children from school. People in the community would refuse to sit by him. Ryan eventually moved to a new community in Indiana and attended a high school where he was warmly accepted.

The Ryan White story made news around the world. Ryan appeared on several television shows and in news magazines and newspapers. He fought for the rights of those with HIV and AIDS and was viewed as a hero in the HIV community. He urged the need for compassion and the importance of removing the stigma associated with the infection. Though he was not the only person with AIDS facing these challenges, he became the voice of many because he was a "socially acceptable" symbol of the disease in the early years of the epidemic. He befriended celebrities and politicians.

In 1988, four years after his diagnosis, Ryan gave testimony to the National Commission on AIDS and spoke at the National Education Association meeting. In his testimony, Ryan told the committee of his experience as a hemophiliac, and later learning that he had AIDS. He described the discrimination he faced, as well as the financial and emotional hardships his family faced. He maintained that he had no hatred for those who treated him badly, because he felt that they were "victims of their own ignorance." He stressed the importance of education regarding HIV and AIDS, because that made all the difference in his new community, where he excelled as a student and was socially accepted.

In 1990, the year that Ryan White died, the U.S. Congress enacted the Ryan White CARE Act. The CARE Act helps communities meet the varied needs of those infected with HIV, such as emergency relief funding, health care and support services, and AIDS education training programs. Each year the Ryan White National Youth Conference is held for young AIDS activists, with the goal of enhancing their leadership and advocacy skills and providing strategies and models for improving HIV prevention. Ryan's mother has made it her mission to continue her son's legacy by speaking across the country against the intolerance and stigma encountered by those with HIV and AIDS. She has played a key role in the preservation of the Ryan White CARE Act and HIV prevention programs.

MAGIC JOHNSON: THE ICON OF "LIVING WELL" WITH HIV

Five-time National NBA Champion, nine-time All-NBA First Team, three-time league Most Valuable Player, and Olympic Gold medalist, Earvin "Magic" Johnson shocked the world in 1991 when he announced he was HIV-positive. In his speech, he attempted to clear up the erroneous beliefs that people held about HIV by stating that HIV/AIDS was not a "gay person's disease." He brought attention to the growing epidemic among heterosexuals and minority communities.

Though Johnson retired in 1991 in light of his diagnosis, he returned to the NBA a year later for a brief comeback, and, not unlike Ryan White, he faced ignorance and discrimination. Some players refused to play basketball with Johnson due to their fear of becoming infected. This provided Johnson with the opportunity to educate the public and the sports world about HIV/AIDS. He says he had to let everyone know, "You couldn't get it by playing basketball against me or high fiving me or hugging me." Johnson also presented the public with a new face of HIV. He appeared healthy and continued to be physically active due to early and effective treatment with antiretroviral therapy. Johnson maintained that it was difficult to accept his HIV status initially, but with the support of his family, education about the disease, and perpetuation of a positive attitude, he has managed to live a normal life.

In 1991, Johnson founded the Magic Johnson Foundation, which "works to develop programs and support community-based organizations that address the educational, health, and social needs of ethnically diverse, urban communities." The foundation has given over $1 million to programs within communities that focus on HIV/AIDS education and prevention. It has also partnered with Abbott Laboratories, an international health-care company, to create the Campaign to End Black HIV/AIDS as a part of the "I Stand With Magic" program. The program focuses on HIV education and awareness, HIV prevention, the importance of regular testing, and current treatments for HIV. The campaign's goal is to cut the rate of new infections among blacks by half by the year 2012.

Johnson speaks regularly to young people across the country about his story and the importance of HIV education and prevention. He tells teenagers how he contracted HIV through unprotected sex, and about the challenges he faced, what he has learned from the experience, and how he has managed to sustain his health. Magic Johnson has given AIDS a new face in the public eye: one that is healthy, strong, and courageous.

Magic Johnson's story changed the way HIV/AIDS was viewed throughout the country, especially in the black community. The period following Johnson's disclosure was marked by increased awareness of HIV/AIDS and open discussions regarding the disease. Testing rates increased in some areas, and several public education and prevention campaigns were launched by organizations and other celebrities. Unfortunately, some feel the enthusiasm was short-lived. The rate of new infections continued to rise among urban and minority populations. The Magic Johnson Foundation's message from the chairman states, "There are still too many people not receiving adequate treatment and care for HIV/AIDS..."

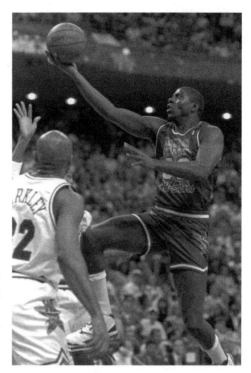

Figure 8.1 West guard Magic Johnson goes for a layup during first-quarter action in the NBA All-Star game at the Orlando Arena in Orlando, Florida, 1992. (AP/Wide World Photos)

GLOBAL HEALTH EFFECT

In 2007, there were an estimated 33.2 million people living with HIV and an estimated 2.1 million deaths from HIV around the world. With an estimated 2.5 million new infections in 2007, HIV continues to make a drastic impact on the global community. Each country has its own unique profile regarding highest-risk populations and the most common mode of transmission; however, the effects of this disease continue to affect the whole world.

Orphan Crisis

It is estimated that 15 million children have been orphaned worldwide due to the loss of one or both of their parents to AIDS. The region hardest hit by this orphan crisis (and HIV in general) is sub-Saharan Africa. It is estimated that the number of children orphaned by AIDS will continue to rise for another decade or two.

The children orphaned by AIDS usually reside with family members or a surviving parent, but others are placed in orphanages or designated housing or live on the street, often in substandard conditions. These children are commonly neglected, abused, and taken advantage of. Some of them are forced to separate from their siblings. They are often stigmatized even if they themselves do not have HIV infection. It is sometimes assumed that the child is also infected with HIV regardless of their actual status, and this further isolates the child from society. They may be denied access to school or normal social activities.

Children growing up in such unstable environments often suffer considerable psychological distress, having lost one or both parents to this illness at a young age. In some towns, the death rate from AIDS is so high that coffin shops are commonly found in shopping districts. Funeral songs may be frequently heard as family and friends walk in a procession for their lost loved one. Children may come to view their own village as a place where AIDS has taken a huge toll and death is frequent.

Children orphaned by AIDS also face difficulties receiving an education for several reasons. Some cannot afford uniforms for school. Others have to stay home to take care of their siblings or work in order to contribute to expenses at home. Other children are required to relocate frequently, making it difficulty to attend a school consistently and establish friendships. Some children may turn to high-risk behavior out of desperation or need for attention, such as criminal activity, or exchanging sexual favors for money.

The orphan crisis has affected family structures throughout sub-Saharan countries. With the lack of parents, boys and girls are not provided with an opportunity to observe their parents as role models. They do not have the opportunity to participate in bonding experiences with their parents and often lack a well-balanced upbringing and socialization. Some miss out on things as common as learning to cook, clean, play sports, or eat properly. When these children become adults, they may not be prepared to become involved in relationships or parent their own children.

Because HIV most commonly affects young adults (i.e., of reproductive age), the epidemic has led to many deaths in this demographic group, leaving a disproportionate number of children and grandparents, both traditionally sectors of society that depend on young adults for support. Because young adults also comprise the bulk of the work force, the toll incurred from HIV-related illnesses and deaths in this demographic group has dramatically affected availability of teachers, doctors, and other professionals. This has resulted not only in a significant economic impact, particularly in underdeveloped countries, but also in a diminished capacity to fight the epidemic through educational preventive efforts and medical interventions.

ECONOMIC EFFECT

Treatment and prevention of HIV was estimated to cost approximately $14 billion per year worldwide in 2007, but this is a small portion of the economic impact that the epidemic of HIV/AIDS has had on the world. The cost of the disease goes far beyond treatment and prevention. It extends to the household, the workplace, the government, and the international community. Research on the economic effect of HIV/AIDS is limited by its immense scope and the interaction of multiple variable factors, but has led to some estimates in small studies.

Let's start with the household. If there is one or more person within a household infected with HIV, that person would need to make regular visits to the doctor and have regular blood tests performed. Time lost from work to attend doctor visits and the cost of transportation to and from the visits, neither of which is trivial in many countries, is often underappreciated. If someone becomes ill and requires hospitalization, that is more time away from work, which results in decreased pay. This can place HIV-positive parents or guardians in a position that would make it difficult to provide food and shelter for their families. Surveys of households that included an HIV-positive member in South Africa in 2002 showed nearly half of the families did not have enough food to feed their children. Not only are families losing money because a provider is unable to work, but families must also pay for funeral costs (often years before the national life expectancy average), which can also be a serious expense. In countries like those in southern Africa, where death from HIV is common and can occur in the same family more than once, this can be a significant financial burden.

What about the other side of the story? If an employee cannot come in for work because he is ill or has to leave early because he is ill, the employer also loses money. This is called loss of productivity, because the person is not at work to produce the goods or services that the company sells/provides. This may seem small if it involves one person, but imagine the impact of millions. The total effect of HIV/AIDS has been difficult to predict due to the complexity of the disease. However, studies predict that AIDS will slow economic growth mainly due to its impact on human resources. This not only affects large production companies, but it also affects schools, hospitals, and other trades. In Kenya, schools were forced to close in 1998 because the country was losing an average of 18 teachers per day to AIDS. Jobs like teaching, which require training, are associated with additional financial losses due to HIV, because there is a cost to train another individual for the job. As more people must be trained to replace those who fall terminally ill from AIDS, costs escalate. This is further complicated by the fact that, as previously discussed, the age group that is being most severely affected by HIV is 18 to 49, the working population.

Unfortunately the costs of HIV do not end at the level of business interactions; they also spill over into governmental economics. With a decrease in the number of teachers, there is an impact on the education that children receive, which affects the jobs they can get. This results in a reduction in the number of qualified individuals to fill the roles of government leaders, college professors, engineers, doctors, and so on, which potentially leaves the country with poor leaders, bad roads, a poor health-care system, and a high level of underemployment. In addition, the decrease in overall national production of consumer goods reduces the country's ability to trade with other countries. As a result, the country loses money by either having to buy more products from other countries or by not being able to sell enough of their products to other countries. This disadvantage particularly affects countries such as Tanzania and Malawi, where the population depends on farming of cash crops.

POPULATION EFFECT

The AIDS epidemic has affected virtually every country in the world, caused more than 25 million deaths since the beginning of the epidemic, and nearly 40 million people are estimated to be living with HIV around the world. The burden of this disease on the global population is immense. Though treatments are available, they are only accessible to a fraction of all infected persons, and there are still millions of people dying of AIDS each year. The World Health Organization estimates that there are millions of people who need antiretroviral therapy that don't have access to these medications (Table 8.1).

Infection rates are still increasing in countries such as Russia, Ukraine, China, India, and others. Although the life expectancy in the United States for persons who are HIV positive has increased dramatically, in some countries in southern Africa that are severely affected by the disease, it is estimated that the average life expectancy has decreased by 16 years due to HIV infection. Other countries that are expected to see a drop in life expectancy are the Bahamas, Cambodia, Dominican Republic, Haiti, and Myanmar. If worldwide distribution of antiretroviral drug therapy can be successfully accomplished, it is estimated that the life expectancy will recover by 2020.

As we discussed, the age group suffering the most from HIV/AIDS around the world is ages 18 to 49, the working and childbearing population. Three-fourths

Table 8.1 Antiretroviral Therapy in Low- and Middle-income Countries by Region, December 2009

Estimated number of adults and children (combined) receiving antiretroviral therapy and needing antiretroviral therapy and percentage coverage in low- and middle-income countries by region, December 2003 to December 2008[a]

Geographical region	Estimated number of people receiving antiretroviral therapy, December 2008 [range]	Estimated number of people needing antiretroviral therapy, 2008 [range][a]	Antiretroviral therapy coverage, December 2008 [range][a]	Estimated number of people receiving antiretroviral therapy, December 2007 [range]	Estimated number of people needing antiretroviral therapy, 2007 [range][a]	Antiretroviral therapy coverage, December 2007 [range][b]	Estimated number of people receiving antiretroviral therapy, December 2003 [range]
Sub-Saharan Africa	2 925 000 [2 690 000–3 160 000]	6 700 000 [6 100 000–7 100 000]	44% [41–48%]	2 100 000 [1 905 000–2 295 000]	6 400 000 [5 900 000–7 000 000]	33% [30–36%]	100 000 [75 000–125 000]
Eastern and Southern Africa	2 395 000 [2 205 000–2 585 000]	5 000 000 [4 500 000–5 300 000]	48% [45–53%]	1 680 000 [1 550 000–1 810 000]	4 700 000 [4 300 000–5 200 000]	36% [33–39%]	75 000 [56 000–94 000]
Western and Central Africa	530 000 [485 000–575 000]	1 800 000 [1 500 000–1 900 000]	30% [28–34%]	420 000 [360 000–480 000]	1 700 000 [1 500 000–1 900 000]	25% [22–28%]	25 000 [19 000–31 000]
Latin America and the Caribbean	445 000 [405 000–485 000]	820 000 [750 000–870 000]	54% [51–60%]	390 000 [350 000–430 000]	770 000 [700 000–820 000]	50% [47–55%]	210 000 [160 000–260 000]
Latin America	405 000 [370 000–440 000]	740 000 [680 000–790 000]	55% [52–60%]	360 000 [320 000–400 000]	700 000 [640 000–750 000]	51% [47–56%]	206 000 [156 000–255 000]
Caribbean	40 000 [35 000–45 000]	75 000 [66 000–83 000]	51% [46–59%]	30 000 [25 000–35 000]	70 000 [61 000–80 000]	43% [37–49%]	4 000 [3 000–5 000]
East, South and South-East Asia	565 000 [520 000–610 000]	1 500 000 [1 200 000–1 900 000]	37% [31–47%]	420 000 [375 000–465 000]	1 500 000 [1 100 000–1 800 000]	29% [23–37%]	70 000 [52 000–88 000]
Europe and Central Asia	85 000 [80 000–90 000]	370 000 [330 000–450 000]	23% [19–27%]	54 000 [51 000–57 000]	340 000 [280 000–410 000]	16% [13–19%]	15 000 [11 000–19 000]
North Africa and the Middle East	10 000 [9 000–11 000]	68 000 [52 000–90 000]	14% [11–19%]	7 000 [6 000–8 000]	63 000 [48 000–86 000]	11% [8–14%]	1 000 [750–1 250]
Total	**4 030 000** [3 700 000–4 360 000]	**9 500 000** [8 600 000–10 000 000]	**42%** [40–47%]	**2 970 000** [2 680 000–3 260 000]	**9 000 000** [8 200 000–9 900 000]	**33%** [30–36%]	**400 000** [300 000–500 000]

Note: some numbers do not add up due to rounding.

[a] For an explanation of the methods used see explanatory notes for Annex 1. See Box 4.2 on estimating treatment need for an interpretation of the data on antiretroviral therapy need and coverage in 2007 and 2008.

[b] The coverage estimate is based on the unrounded estimated numbers of people receiving and needing antiretroviral therapy.

Source: Towards universal access: Scaling up priority HIV/AIDS interventions in the health sector. Progress report 2010 (WHO, UNICEF, UNAIDS).

of the AIDS-related deaths in southern Africa have been within this age group. Among this group, women are the most vulnerable to new infections. The disruptions to the family structure and the workforce have had a dramatic impact on the local communities.

BARRIERS TO TREATMENT

The burden of HIV/AIDS has continued to afflict the world despite the availability (in some countries) of multiple treatment options. Deaths from AIDS around the world continue to occur as a result of multiple obstacles to treatment and high quality health-care services. We can think of these obstacles in two categories: individual barriers and structural barriers.

Individual Barriers

The individual barriers to treatment that HIV-positive persons face include limited access to care, stigma, and personal or cultural beliefs. These barriers are shared by HIV-positive people in rich and poor countries. "Limited access" refers to the inability or near-inability for individuals to receive health-care services. This may be due to failure to find a nearby clinic or physician, for example in rural areas where there may be few physicians available. In urban areas, physicians and clinics may be overbooked. Visits to the doctor also may require individuals to take time off from work and arrange transportation, extra costs that some individuals cannot afford.

Though there is a great quantity of information about HIV and AIDS available to the public, stigma and mistaken beliefs regarding HIV and AIDS persist. The shame surrounding HIV still exists and can result in denial of obvious symptoms. The latest prevention campaigns encourage knowledge and disclosure of HIV status between individuals who plan to engage in activity that put either person at risk of transmission, such as sexual intercourse or drug use, but such disclosures are not necessarily routine. Individuals at risk who are tested regularly and diagnosed early in the course of infection may seek treatment earlier in the course of disease, as opposed to delaying seeking medical attention until the disease has reached a point in which it is much harder to effectively control. Unfortunately, studies suggest that patients are still being diagnosed relatively late in the course of infection, when their CD4 counts are already dangerously low. At this point, health-care costs for the more significant complications of advanced disease are much higher and the likelihood of success in controlling HIV infection is less and less the later the patient presents for care.

Structural Barriers

The structural barriers are more frequently encountered by developing countries, though these barriers exist in parts of the United States and other wealthier nations as well. Poor communication and transportation systems are critical barriers to HIV treatment. Bad roads and lack of public transportation make it difficult for individual to go to their nearest clinic, which is usually miles away from home. Limited health-care facilities and staff result in crowded clinics and overworked staff. Patients may be forced to leave and return to the clinic on another day because they can not be seen or because they can not afford to wait for hours due to work or other commitments. The staff may also be undereducated due to high demand, high turnover due to HIV-related deaths, and rushed training. Decentralization of care, for example between the public and private sector, or between different clinics that do not communicate with each other, results in the absence of a single cohesive medical record, treatment plan, or educational program for each individual. Patients can get easily lost within such systems. Even when clinics are relatively well-established for treatment there may be inadequate medical infrastructure to support safety laboratory testing, follow up assessments, and management of complications.

Countries also face treatment barriers due to job instability and poverty, which fuel food insecurity and constant migration. Some people who have difficulty finding work are forced to move from place to place just to feed themselves or their families. It becomes difficult to find another primary HIV doctor in each new location, and to coordinate their health care. This results in fragmented care, potential lapses in treatment, and/or possible lack of adherence to a medication regimen. Some patients simply can't afford HIV medications, especially in countries where drug assistance programs don't exist. Lack of job stability and poverty also give rise to lack of fundamental resources such as food and shelter. These needs often become a priority over medical care. This can be harmful to individuals with HIV or AIDS because their immune system is weakened and put at further risk by poor nutrition, hygiene, or access to medical care, but they may feel forced to choose work over health care, or paying for food over paying for medications.

SUMMARY

HIV has had a tremendous impact on the health-care system and society as a whole, affecting every aspect of society within the United States and throughout the world. There have been many victories in the fight against HIV and AIDS over the last 25 years, but there are still substantial challenges. HIV continues to kill millions of people each year despite the availability of treatment. Because of its far-reaching social, economic, and global effects, HIV is a disease that affects everyone. As history tells us, it is only injurious to separate ourselves from the epidemic. Rather, it is important to protect ourselves and educate others about the disease. Public icons like Ryan White and Magic Johnson have paved the way for heroic acts of courage and reshaping the public vision of this illness, but more work remains to be done.

9

Lessons Learned and Future Directions

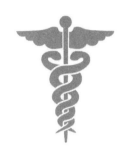

Sigall K. Bell, MD

This chapter reviews the last quarter-century of HIV: how far have we come during this time and what directions do we need to focus on now? We will answer the following questions:

- What are some of the successes of the last 25 years of HIV care?
- What are some of the failures?
- Why has vaccine development been so challenging?
- What are some other research priorities?

Over a quarter-century has elapsed since cases of what became known as HIV were first described in 1981. Three decades later, there have been some remarkable successes but also some notable setbacks. What have we learned during this time and how does it shape our next steps moving forward?

SUCCESSES

Discovery

The early years of the HIV epidemic were marked by scientific inquiry and discovery. Doctors and scientists worked hard to identify the virus, and to develop a test to detect HIV. We have learned a lot about how HIV infects cells, replicates, and causes damage to the immune system. We have also learned about its ability to remain dormant and "hide" in some cells, resulting in important implications for goals of treatment. By understanding the key mechanisms of transmission, we were able to begin to take strides toward prevention of HIV infection.

Pathogenesis

Imagine an impending train wreck: a speeding train is about to go over a cliff. Untreated HIV infection has been likened to this scenario: the CD4 count represents the length of remaining track before the train goes over the cliff. The viral load represents the speed of the train. The goal of treatment is to prevent the train from going over the cliff. Medications can do this by significantly increasing the CD4 count (lengthening the tracks) and by slowing down the train, in some cases nearly to a halt, by reducing the viral load.

In chapter 6 we discussed the concept of the viral set point. Early HIV studies have shown us that the viral set point is an important determinant of the pace of HIV progression. We have learned that there are several factors that affect the viral load. These include viral factors and host (or human) factors. The key viral factor is aggressiveness of the particular strain of infecting virus. Some viruses are more aggressive than others because they replicate more quickly. Others are much weaker.

Several host factors also affect disease progression. One example is genetic factors. In the same way that people have different blood types, we also have different human leukocyte antigen (HLA) types. HLA serves many important functions, including defense from infections, protection against cancers, and a role in some autoimmune diseases. You may have heard of these important molecules in the context of organ transplantation. When someone gets a transplant, doctors try to match the HLA of the recipient and the donor as closely as possible to prevent rejection of the transplanted organ.

When a human cell is infected by a virus, the cell breaks down the viral particles and presents special viral particles on HLA class I molecules on its surface. These particles on the HLA molecules serve as flags for the immune system. They tell the body that the cell bearing the flag has been infected and is therefore a target for destruction. Scientists have found that certain HLA molecules make it more likely that HIV will progress more quickly, while others predict a slower disease course.

In addition, some people have a genetic factor that make their T cells more resistant to HIV infection. This factor—the CCR5 deletion—is a change in the

CCR5 human coreceptor (which HIV uses to enter the cell). We introduced the concept of the CCR5 mutation in chapter 2. Persons who are homozygous, or have two copies of the altered CCR5 receptor gene, are much less likely to get ill from HIV.

Finally, there are many human factors that are not inherited, but that rather arise in response to HIV infection. These acquired factors also affect disease progression. For example, the strength and breadth of the host immune response to HIV also predict how well the individual will be able to control the infection.

Researchers have found several important immune markers in persons with HIV who have very slow disease progression. Several terms have been used to describe this unique group of persons, including long-term nonprogressors, controllers, or elite controllers—a rare group of people that have HIV but control the virus to undetectable levels by conventional testing in the absence of HIV medications. Scientists hope that by studying such unique individuals we can learn about the critical components to controlling the virus—the so called immune correlates of protection from HIV progression. Studies so far have found that different components of the immune system may each play a role, including T lymphocytes, neutralizing antibodies (which neutralize HIV by targeting and attacking it effectively), and Natural Killer cells (part of the innate human immune system).

Diagnostic Testing

A sensitive and specific test to diagnose HIV has been instrumental to linking people with treatment and preventing further transmission of HIV. Over the years, tests have become more efficient and less expensive. New tests like "rapid HIV tests," which can be done right on the spot from a drop of blood or even a saliva swab, have been helpful additions to our testing strategies in testing centers, emergency rooms, or urgent care centers. This approach helps to avoid "loss to follow up"—the problem that occurs when people are tested with a blood sample that has to be sent to the lab (and results that become available several days later) but then don't return to get their results, never learning if the test was positive. Finally, in combination with viral load testing, the development of resistance testing (although still expensive and not readily available everywhere) has helped doctors fortunate to access this tool to design the most effective possible medication regimen to control the virus.

Drug Development

The development of individual HIV drugs has also been an important success story of the last quarter-century. Activists worked hard to apply pressure to hasten

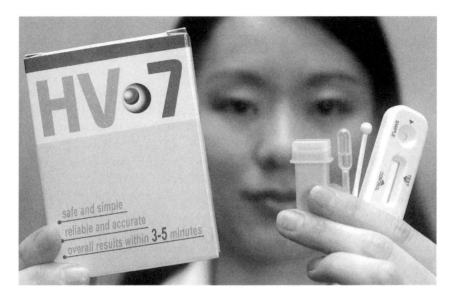

Figure 9.1 A woman shows HV-7, said to be the first world's fastest HIV rapid test kit in 2004. The HV-7 rapid test kit was developed for increased efficiency of diagnosis and a means to connect positive individuals to care at the point of testing. (AP/ Wide World Photos)

the process of drug testing and development in order to release medications for use as soon as possible. This too was a life-saving maneuver, since people who acquired HIV in the early part of the epidemic were first treated with just one or two drugs and rapidly developed resistance to these medications and others in the same class of drugs. The new medicines were essential to fight the resistant virus. Over the 25 years since illnesses that were later discovered to be HIV were described, approximately 25 drugs have been developed and approved for use, providing new options for individuals with difficult-to-treat infections.

Better Medications

Other benefits to the robust development of new drugs are improved "pill burden" and side-effect profile. Instead of having to take a handful of pills every several hours (historically leading patients to set alarm clocks to remember their pills several times a day), persons with HIV infection now have the potential option of taking just one pill once a day, thanks to medication advances that allow three drugs to be packaged into one pill. This makes it easier for people to remember to take their medicines. It also makes the treatment of HIV less intrusive in people's daily lives, since regimens don't typically dominate a patient's daily activities. The HIV medications have also been improved to eliminate some of the undesirable side effects, making them easier to take.

Increased Survival

Once a fatal disease, HIV is now largely viewed as a manageable chronic illness in countries with access to effective antiretroviral medication, as long as individuals with HIV take their medications regularly. This fact is single-handedly the most remarkable medical success of HIV care in the last 25 years. The advent of highly active antiretroviral therapy has saved many lives in those countries where it is readily available.

SETBACKS

Despite these important advances in HIV recognition and treatment, there are a few areas that have not come as far as we hoped in the last 25 years. Although the stigma of HIV infection is slowly decreasing in some areas, many people still suffer from it. While we have new tools to diagnose and treat HIV, they are not reaching everyone who would benefit from them, and many lives that could be saved are lost because not everyone can access antiretroviral therapy. Although we have come a long way in controlling HIV, we have not found a cure. By identifying failures of the last quarter-century, we can help sharpen our focus on areas that need our attention in the coming years.

Case Identification

Across the world, voluntary counseling and testing centers have opened their doors to help people gain access to HIV testing. Education programs have also been developed globally to teach people about the virus, its mechanisms of transmission, and the kinds of health problems it can cause. Yet there are still many people who have HIV that don't know they are infected. The CDC estimate that one-quarter of the U.S. cases are undiagnosed is appalling. This figure is likely to be even larger on a global scale. Armed with better, rapid tests and education programs, we need to do a better job at identifying undiagnosed cases so that those persons can be linked to appropriate care and avoid further transmission of HIV.

Late Presentation

Studies suggest that the average CD4 count at the time of diagnosis is dangerously low. This means that we are missing the opportunity to catch people who are living with HIV earlier in their course, so that damage to the immune system can be prevented. In addition to having important implications for individual patients by avoiding a dangerous decline in their health status, earlier diagnosis can also help our health-care system by avoiding the much larger costs associated with treating people who have more advanced disease problems, and by preventing "unknowing" spread of the virus to other people. The need for earlier diagnosis points back to a broader reach on screening efforts, including an active attempt to institute universal screening.

Education and Prevention

The number of new infections in the United States each year has not dropped significantly over several years despite widespread education and counseling programs. This suggests that there aren't enough programs, they aren't reaching the highest-risk populations, or they just aren't effective enough—all areas that need priority attention.

Global Treatment Programs

Although drug development has been a success story in the United States, the availability of drugs on a global scale has been a relative failure. The World Health Organization launched an ambitious "3 by 5" program, aiming to get three million HIV-positive persons on treatment by 2005. This effort highlighted some of the challenges in delivering medications worldwide, since it fell short of its goal. Many people see this as a humanitarian crisis, since the lack of medication availability worldwide means that people who could have been saved are dying every day. Subsequent effects of this dramatic death toll are also harrowing problems, including collapse of the work force and an orphan crisis in some countries that have been hit particularly hard by this epidemic.

Global treatment programs require considerable financial investment, cooperation from pharmaceutical companies, political willpower and commitment, and a stable health-care infrastructure to facilitate treatment implementation and monitoring of potentially harmful side effects and treatment failures. Each of these areas needs further attention and support.

Vaccine Development

Despite vigorous research efforts, the development of a vaccine to prevent HIV infection has escaped our reach over the last quarter-century. The virus has proven to be particularly clever and "out-smarts" vaccines to date.

Think about some of the vaccines you have gotten over your lifetime: measles, mumps, rubella, tetanus, and others. Vaccines usually work by "showing" the immune system part of the disease and allowing it to form a protective antibody against that disease. In the case of measles, for example, the body forms an antibody to an inactivated measles virus. In the case of tetanus, the body forms an antibody to a modified protein toxin produced by the bacteria that causes tetanus. Why is it so difficult to develop a vaccine against HIV?

One secret to HIV's ability to evade vaccines is its reverse transcriptase enzyme. Remember in chapter 2 we discussed that this enzyme is error-prone, and that the mistakes it makes in replicating the HIV genome provide the virus with opportunities to develop mutations. Sometimes these mutations can work in the virus's favor. The viral genome encodes the necessary proteins to make new virus. A mistake in replication of the virus's genetic material can change the size or shape of one of its proteins. This happens because amino acids, the building blocks that make up proteins, all come in different shapes and sizes. Imagine, for example, that a mistake in replication changes the genetic code to one that replaces a small amino acid A with a bulky amino acid B on a chain of amino acids that make up a viral protein. Let's also imagine that the body typically recognizes this particular protein by binding it with a neutralizing antibody at the site of amino acid A. Now that amino acid A has been replaced by amino acid B, the neutralizing antibody no longer recognizes it and it is not flagged for destruction. We say that the virus has "escaped" from immune control because bulky amino acid B looks different and maybe doesn't even fit into the binding groove of the antibody that was supposed to detect the viral protein.

The most encouraging vaccine trial results so far came from a large study in Thailand. Over 16,000 individuals were randomized to receive either a vaccine (comprised of two different HIV vaccines) or placebo. Over three years of follow-up there were 56 new HIV infections in the vaccine group, compared to 76 infections in the placebo group, which was found to be statistically significant. Still, it isn't clear which of these two vaccines was most important (and what the actual "immune correlates" of control really were), and whether the duration of protection will hold over time. The vaccine also wasn't fully protective, in that a significant number of infections still occurred.

Thought Box

Viral escape from immune control has been one big limiting factor in developing an enduring vaccine. Imagine what it would be like if you were trying to catch someone who moved quickly and kept changing his or her clothes. It would be hard to recognize your target. How can scientists catch something that keeps changing its appearance?

SUMMARY

The last quarter-century has been marked by notable successes in HIV care but has also provided some important lessons about areas of focus that need more attention. Among the greatest successes are improved medications and dramatically increased survival of HIV-infected persons. Among the failures are inadequate global treatment roll-out programs and the inability to develop, so far, a vaccine that is highly effective in preventing HIV acquisition. Developing a vaccine has been particularly challenging because of HIV's clever way of "changing its appearance" so that it can evade the immune system. These areas help to shape our research and treatment priorities moving forward.

10

"My Story"

Sigall K. Bell, MD

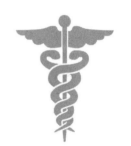

This chapter showcases three real life stories about HIV written by patients with this illness. Until now, we have talked mostly about the scientific, medical, or social views about HIV infection. What do people living with HIV have to say about their own experience of illness? Sometimes the most powerful lessons we can learn about medicine come from the patients themselves. Here are three stories to consider from Judy, John, and Christopher. As you read them, think about the following questions for discussion:

1. Did Judy, John, or Christopher experience stigma as part of their experience with HIV? What was it like?
2. How do you think HIV changed each of their lives? Socially? Spiritually? Physically? Mentally?
3. What medical complications of HIV can you recognize in their stories?
4. What, if anything, do you think would be different about their stories if they unfolded today?
5. What questions would you want to ask Judy, John, or Christopher if you had the chance?

JUDY'S STORY

Living positive with HIV has become one of the pillars that holds up my life. I was diagnosed with HIV in 1990, when I was living in South Africa. In those days, essentially all that anyone knew about AIDS was that it was a death sentence: you might live for a few years after getting the virus, but you would get sicker and sicker, and that was that.

In 1990 I was 39 years old, had two kids from a previous marriage, and worked as an artist. Like so many women who get HIV, I probably got the infection from a partner whom I lived with for years, in a long and loving relationship. My crash course in the virus came after my partner was hospitalized with HIV, and I went for a test. He died three years later. At that time, there was no medicine available to us that worked against the HIV virus.

But I was lucky. In the late 1990s, around the time I started to get really ill, medical science found combinations of antiretrovirals that control the virus, so that a person can live a long and healthy life with HIV. My family encouraged me to come home to Boston, where I got treatment.

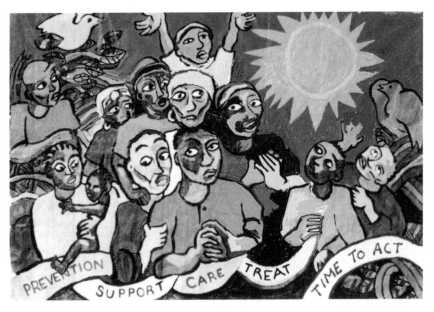

Figure 10.1 *Time to Act,* banner, Judy Seidman, painted in 1994. (Courtesy of Judy Ann Seidman)

The medicine works. I went from being hospitalized with HIV and meningitis due to tuberculosis (TB) to getting on with a normal, working life. I have lived to see my kids grow up and have lives of their own, and my parents grow old. I will be 60 in June. I still have the virus.

And I learned a serious lesson: people can only help you if they know that you need help. Yes, each of us has a right to privacy about our medical condition, and there is still a lot of stigma about HIV and AIDS. Many people still think you get HIV because you did something wrong. It is hard to say out loud: I have this problem, this condition. But none of us can survive alone, without people who care for you.

A friend of mine said: we should tell everyone who is HIV positive to list 10 fantastic, wonderful things that happened to you after you were diagnosed. And

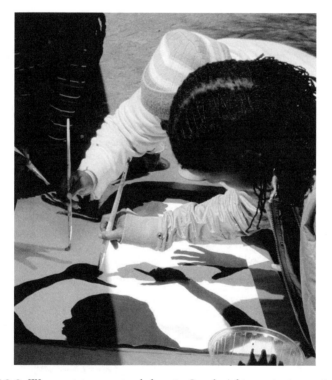

Figure 10.2 Women in an art workshop in South Africa painting a picture that they later titled "Women Working Together Can Turn the World Right-Side Up." (Courtesy of Judy Ann Seidman)

you will be amazed to discover that there are 10 really wonderful things since you found out you had this thing.

So today, sometimes I paint pictures about what it means to live with this virus and in a world with this epidemic—as well as about all the other things that I see around me. My 10 most wonderful things get expressed in color, when I make art and celebrate life. I teach art-making in workshops, looking at the problems and hopes that each of us finds in our daily lives, as individuals and as members of our community. The AIDS epidemic is part of that fabric; we use drawing and color and shape and line to explore how this virus is part of our lives; and how we, together, make our lives and the lives of people we care for, better

We paint pictures that tell how we can fight and win against this thing we call AIDS, and this struggle becomes a positive part of our stories.

Judy

JOHN'S STORY

Life was full of promise for me back in the early 1980s. I had a great job in the travel industry and got to see many parts of the world. I also met my life companion in 1980. Neither of us had been promiscuous, and we felt that we were safe from the ever-increasing news about the HIV virus and AIDS epidemic. He was divorced, had one adult child, and had just come out of a three-year relationship with another man. He was also a very talented man; a master tailor from Portugal, an artist, and a musician. He was caring and giving, besides being a very handsome man as well.

We moved in together after a year of seeing each other and opened up a tailor shop and sold custom men's and ladies' suits. I still worked in the travel industry and did the bookkeeping for the shop and handled the customers on the very busy weekends. The business took off and we were able to move closer to work and buy our first home. We vacationed in Portugal, and on one visit we were able to purchase an ocean front lot and eventually build a vacation/retirement home there. Life couldn't be better.

One day in early 1990 my companion wasn't feeling well, which was very unlike him. He had a flu-like infection with the cough and fever and chills and after seeing our primary care physician was placed on antibiotics. I remember him saying that it was the first time he had ever had to take anything stronger than an aspirin. It took forever for him to clear that up, but when it finally went away I noticed a change in skin color on his cheek. It was a small, dark discoloration but I told him he should get it checked out with a dermatologist. The dermatologist removed the growth and sent it out for testing and at the same time told him that he was should get some blood tests including the test for the AIDS virus.

He came home and told me what had transpired and we were both upset but confident that it was just a routine safety measure and would be no problem; after all we had been together for 10 years. It took a week for the test results to come back. It was one of the scariest waiting periods of my life. Finally the day came and results were in, positive for the HIV virus, and the test of his skin growth came back as positive for Kaposi sarcoma (KS) at the same time. We were devastated. I felt like I was hit by a truck and handed our death certificates at the same time. We cried a lot, hugged a lot, reminded each other how much we loved each other but together decided that we could beat this thing. He was given the name of an infectious disease doctor and an appointment was made. I went with him. The doctor said that he was going to test me for the virus, and another week of anxiety followed. Mine also came back positive as I suspected it would.

The only medication that could "slow the progression" at the time was AZT, which was prescribed once every six hours around the clock, as well as chemotherapy for my companion to treat the KS. That meant setting the alarm to wake us up at night to take the AZT dose and going to chemo three times a week. We saw a holistic doctor and took various types of supplements, hoping to make a difference. We listened to the news about any new advances in the fight against HIV and read as much as we could about the right things to do. We were paying our own life and health insurance at the time, as well as two auto loans and two mortgages, and the usual business expenses at the shop.

We decided to keep the diagnosis a secret from our families. This we did until the spring of 1993. My companion's condition worsened, and by this time we had to close the shop and I had to leave work to care for him at home. Neighbors shunned us and wouldn't even say hello if we happened to meet in the yard. We never told them but they suspected.

We had already started to cut back on contact with family and friends at this point and wouldn't return calls or visit. We isolated ourselves. The medical insurance costs were rising, and the medications costs were soaring to the point that our retirement home had to be sold, a car had to be sold, and furnishings in the house had to be sold to meet the cost of the medications and the rising health insurance costs.

I remember my dentist had also moved out of state and recommended another dentist for care. I made an appointment for a six-month check-up and cleaning. He was new in town and did the cleaning himself. I sat in the chair and he put the bib over me. I then asked him if he had received my dental records from my other dentist and he said he had not, and I told him that I was HIV positive. He backed away from the chair and told me to remove the bib and leave and refused to treat me. I was shocked by his reaction and just left, realizing I still had the bib on when I walked into the house and told my companion what had just happened. I felt like I had a giant "A" for AIDS sewn on my shirt.

Finally one day I couldn't take the deep depression I was in any longer and needed to share the burden with someone, and we sat down to discuss who we would tell. My companion phoned his daughter and told her. That was the last phone conversation he ever had with her. I wrote a letter to one of my sisters that I was close with and disclosed the fact that I was HIV positive and my companion was dying. This was in March 1993.

I thank God for a very warm, caring, and loving family that can pull together during a crisis. Without their help I wouldn't have been able to pull through the final days of my companion's life when he passed in July 1993, after 13 years together. My sisters, brothers, and mother would come up and sit with him. His family shunned us. He wasn't the same-looking man as I had met, just a vivid memory. He passed away only 10 days after being placed in a hospice. I will never forget having to call his daughter and my family to tell them the news. I was in deep depression and my family decided to take the reins.

With their help I moved back to Massachusetts and was fortunate enough to find an outstanding primary care physician. Suddenly there were advances in the medications used for HIV, and I am one of the lucky ones to have been able to take part in some of the clinical trials with success. Success with the new "cocktails" has lengthened my life, but the quality has definitely changed. I can no longer work. I am severely thin with muscle wasting and have other problems as well. Food doesn't appeal to me. I try to cook but get "filled up" with the smell of the food and cannot eat it many times. I try to eat what I can when I can.

I have been hospitalized several times with cardiac problems and pneumonia. Initially I felt that some of the nursing staff was ill-at-ease treating a symptomatic HIV patient, but that has changed.

Today I can't keep up with the housework or the yard work. My nephews help out a lot, as do my brothers and sisters. I think soon I may have to move into a place that is easier to care for and on one floor.

Socially I have become asexual as a result of this disease. I do not seek out sex with anyone because of it. I have known many people who have died from this disease over the years from various complications, other than my companion. I often think that if they could have lived a few months longer, they may still be alive because of the advances in research and drugs that occurred shortly, months, after their passing.

I am grateful to be able to be here today, but my life has changed 180 degrees from what it was. I am stared at a lot because I am so painfully thin. I get comments on it from strangers but mostly children. It's the adults I can't forgive. I appear much older than my age and walk slower and generally feel about 20 years older. I am often asked if I want a senior citizen's discount at various stores without being asked for ID. I tell them not quite yet thank you.

Hopefully the newly diagnosed can be able to live a more normal life than I have and, with advances in research, maintain a better quality of life than I have and many older symptomatic HIV patients have. More importantly, with so much information out there now about how to prevent HIV, hopefully the next generation can avoid contracting this illness.

With Life,

John

CHRISTOPHER'S STORY

In September of 1993 during a routine physical examination with my primary care physician, my doctor suggested that I be tested with the so-called AIDS test. At the time I was pretty healthy—on treatment for hypertension but otherwise fine. My doctor was a family friend and confidante, and he was aware of my lifestyle and my relationship with my present-day partner. I agreed to the test and had every belief that it would come back negative.

The next week I received a call at my office from my doctor. The test was positive. He asked me to come in to his office that same day to discuss a course of treatment. When I heard those words at work, I felt like I was in a fog and wasn't even sure I heard him correctly. Even more frightening was the moment I considered how I would break the news to my partner. I immediately called him at work and told him, and all I could hear was him crying on the other end. At that point I could have died—it was just so painful to think about how I had betrayed both him and myself in our relationship.

We met with my doctor shortly thereafter and set up a course of treatment. At that time four pills (two medicines) were taken daily. We waited to see how this would improve my blood tests—my T cell count. This medication regimen kept my counts in an excellent range for few years. But during this time I noticed that my body was physically changing right in front of my eyes. I saw frank muscle wasting, especially in my face and my arms, legs, and buttocks.

At that point I met my HIV doctor, a specialist whom my doctor referred me to in order to get my life and my cells back into order. I was monitored for a three-year period off medication since my T cells were high (and had never been dangerously low even before starting treatment) and the medications seemed to be harming my body—causing painful tingling of my toes and changes in the fat distribution in my body. I knew this was a trial period and that once my T cells began to show signs of dropping again I would need to resume treatment, but at one glorious point I wondered if my body could continue to fight this disease on it own. After a while it was clear that my immune system was not winning the battle. Since some time had passed I had the benefit of going back on medications when the pills were improved—I only had to take one pill once a day in order to gain the benefit of three different drugs that were all wrapped up in one tablet.

On two occasions I had the opportunity to share my story with several student doctors at Harvard Medical School—experiences which were both gratifying and fulfilling for my own therapy. I hoped that by hearing the story of a real human being infected with HIV that the students could feel and see the human element of this disease and begin to learn how to approach the emotional side of this illness with their own future patients. I was really grateful for the chance to tell my story, because it was a major step for me in dealing with the reality of this disease before strangers. At this point, other than a roomful or two of medical students, only my partner knows. Not even my own family is aware of my status, and I cannot say whether I will confide in them about this issue in the near future. I don't want to burden them. Maybe in time I will have the courage to do so, but I don't right now.

More than the disease itself, HIV has taken an emotional toll on both myself and my life partner. If it were not for his love and support, I don't know how I would have gotten through. I am so grateful to have such wonderful medical care and I can't imagine what life would be without my partner's understanding. While things seem to be under control now in terms of my health, whatever comes in the future, both my medical and emotional support will be there to help me get through the next phase. As I expressed to my doctor, there is the element of the "disease" but something worse than the disease itself is the "dis-Ease" of all this that lives in one's mind, and the constant struggle of how to deal with it.

Christopher

11

What You Can Do

Sigall K. Bell, MD

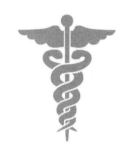

Now that you have had a chance to learn about HIV, what can you do about it? The first step is to be smart about the risk factors for transmission and prevent your own exposure to this illness. If you have had a possible exposure to HIV, talk to a doctor about testing.

If you are moved by the stories in this book about the early days of the HIV epidemic, about some of the trials and tribulations faced by people living with HIV, about Judy's, John's or Christopher's stories, or maybe even those of your own friends or family, you can make a difference. There are many ways to become active in fighting HIV. Some people become health-care providers and help HIV-positive patients. Others become active in their community with many different programs to help HIV-positive people ranging from education to cooking to art to social supports and a host of other activities. You can find out about these online or through your department of public health. You can also find out about HIV/AIDS support groups like AIDS Action and learn about opportunities to contribute. You can ask about programs for HIV-positive patients in your doctor's office or local hospital if you are interested in volunteering. You can reach out by educating your friends and classmates about how to stay safe and when to seek medical attention.

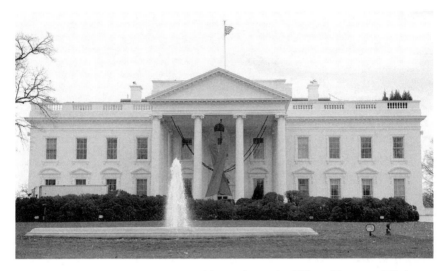

Figure 11.1 An AIDS awareness ribbon adorns the White House in Washington to commemorate World AIDS Day, 2010. (AP/Wide World Photos)

The best way to fight HIV until we can develop an effective vaccine is to increase our awareness, education, prevention, and treatment strategies. Talking about HIV can help us recognize it and prevent its spread.

The problems that have emerged as a result of the global HIV burden are so big that they can seem too overwhelming to address. But each of us can make a difference. HIV can teach us a lot about the power of activism. Because the HIV epidemic started among young and generally disenfranchised populations, it became necessary for the victims of HIV and AIDS to be their own voice. Activist groups became an essential part of the HIV story, because governments and health-care organizations were slower to act. These groups were involved on every front, from increasing public awareness to urging the availability of antiretroviral therapy.

The work of activist groups illustrates the power of the combined voices and actions of the people. There are many groups continuing to work diligently toward prevention of HIV and improvement of quality of life for those living with the virus. These groups, along with government, businesses, and private organizations, are playing a big role in attempts to solve the population and economic consequences of HIV and minimize the barriers to treatment.

If you wish to learn more about HIV/AIDS or get involved in the fight against HIV and AIDS, there are several organizations near you with which you can get involved.

Check out:

Centers for Disease Control and Prevention: http://www.cdc.gov/hiv/
National Institutes of Health: http://www.aidsinfo.nih.gov/
I Stand with Magic: http://www.istandwithmagic.com/
Center for Young Women's Health: http://www.youngwomenshealth.org/
National HIV/AIDS Awareness Days: http://www.hhs.gov/
aidsawarenessdays/

Glossary

Acute retroviral syndrome: A collection of symptoms and signs that often occur when a person is first infected with HIV. These commonly include fever, chills, sweats, sore throat, rash, swollen glands, nausea or vomiting, diarrhea, weight loss, and achy muscles and joints.

Adaptive immunity: A specialized arm of the immune system composed of highly specialized cells and systems that target specific pathogens (invaders). In contrast to innate immunity, adaptive immunity takes longer to activate, but is more specific and powerful.

AIDS: Acquired Immune Deficiency Syndrome (AIDS) is the advanced stage of HIV disease, when the immune system is significantly weakened and/or the CD4 count is less than 200 cells/μL.

AIDS-defining illness: A list of diseases that, when diagnosed in a person infected with HIV, are markers of AIDS.

Anemia: A deficiency of red blood cells that can cause fatigue or weakness.

Antibody: Also called immunoglobulin, this Y-shaped protein is made by B-cells and is used by the immune system to identify and neutralize invaders like bacteria or viruses.

Antigen: A particle that is introduced to the immune system, resulting in the creation of specific antibodies targeting this particle.

Antigen-presenting cells: Specialized cells of the immune system that survey the body and "present" foreign particles (or antigens) on their surface to the other cells in the immune system in order to coordinate and activate a concerted reaction to the pathogen (invader).

Antiretroviral therapy: Medications that target HIV. Used in a combination of at least three drugs, these medications are sometimes also referred to as HAART, or highly active antiretroviral therapy.

AZT: Also called zidovudine or ZDV, this is the first medication (belonging to the nucleoside reverse transcriptase inhibitor, NRTI, class of drugs) that was used to treat HIV.

Basic reproductive rate of infection: Also called basic reproductive number, or basic reproductive ratio, and denoted as R_0, this is an epidemiological term that determines whether an infection will propagate and spread to others or die out. It measures the number of secondary cases that will result from an index case in a population with no immunity to the infection, in the absence of any treatment or intervention.

B cells: Specialized lymphocytes (a type of white blood cell) that are part of the adaptive immune system. These cells make antibodies that target specific antigens (see antigen above).

Capsid: The outer shell of a virus.

CAT scan (or CT scan): Common name for computed tomography scan or dual X-ray computed tomography, a medical imaging technique that allows doctors to see inside the body with three-dimensional images. CAT scan images provide greater detail and resolution than films like X-rays.

CCR5: A receptor on the surface of CD4 cells that is used by HIV to enter the human cell. A small portion of the human population is born with a specific deletion in this receptor, making them more resistant to HIV infections.

CD4 cell: A particular type of T cell (which is a subset of the white blood cells, and also part of the adaptive immune system) named for the CD4 receptor on its cell surface. This is the primary target cell for HIV.

cDNA: "copy" DNA. The DNA that is made from RNA by the enzyme reverse transcriptase. Formation of cDNA is an important step in HIV replication.

Chemotherapeutic agents: Medications used to treat cancer or microorganisms causing infection. Commonly called chemotherapy or chemo, it most commonly refers to cancer-fighting drugs.

Cocktails: The popularized term for highly active antiretroviral therapy. "Cocktails" generally refer to a combination of at least three active antiretroviral drugs.

Cryptococcus: A common fungus that can cause opportunistic infections in immunocompromised people. Cryptococcus can affect several organs in the body, but one common way it is seen in AIDS patients is in the form of an inflammation in the lining of the brain called cryptococcal meningitis.

Cytomegalovirus (CMV): A virus that can cause an opportunistic infection in immunocompromised people. This virus is very common in the general population and generally causes a self-limited illness in healthy individuals. In persons with very low immunity, CMV can reactivate and affect many organs. One such serious complication is called CMV retinitis—when CMV infects the eye.

Dendritic cells: A type of antigen-presenting cell (see antigen-presenting cell). These immune system cells are often present in surfaces that come into contact with the environment, such as skin, the inside of the nose, lungs, and stomach or intestines.

DNA: Deoxyribonucleic acid (DNA) has been called the blueprint of life. It is a nucleic acid that stores all the information and instructions needed to create a new living organism.

Entry inhibitors: A class of HIV medications that prevent entry of HIV into the human cell.

Enzyme-linked immunosorbent assay (ELISA): Also called enzyme immunoassay (EIA), this is a popular biochemical method for diagnostic laboratory testing that detects specific antibodies or antigens. ELISA or EIA testing is the first part in a two-part standard test for HIV. If the HIV ELISA is positive (detecting antibodies to HIV), a second test called the western blot (see western blot) is run. The ELISA is highly sensitive, resulting in few false negative tests. The western blot is highly specific, resulting in few false positives.

Epidemic: An epidemiologic term referring to a condition in which new cases of a certain disease among a specific population during a certain time exceed the expected number of cases. Classic examples include the black death or black plague of the Middle Ages, and the HIV epidemic of the 20th and 21st century. Sometimes the term is used to describe noninfectious diseases, for example the "obesity epidemic." It is also sometimes used interchangeably with pandemic (see pandemic), although this term typically refers to epidemics that have global impact.

Gay-related immune deficiency (GRID): A stigmatizing term used early in the HIV epidemic before the cause of AIDS was known.

Genome: The entire hereditary information of an organism, typically in the form of DNA or RNA.

Hemophilia: A bleeding disorder due to deficiency of an important clotting factor in the blood.

Hepatitis: An inflammation of the liver. Hepatitis A, B, and C are types of viral infections that cause inflammation of the liver.

Highly active antiretroviral therapy (HAART): See antiretroviral therapy.

HIV: Human immunodeficiency virus (HIV) is the virus responsible for HIV disease and ultimately causes AIDS if left untreated.

Human leukocyte antigen (HLA): The human leukocyte antigen system is the name of the major histocompatibility complex in humans, which includes a large number of genes that are involved in immune system function. Each person has a unique set of HLA genes that play an important role in defense against disease, autoimmune disease, and the likelihood of success or rejection of organ transplantation.

Human T-lymphotrophic virus (HTLV): A human RNA retrovirus that causes T cell leukemia and T cell lymphoma. One of the scientific groups to first identify HIV initially named it HTLV-III because of the similarity in structure of HIV to HTLV. Another group that identified HIV called it lymphadenopathy-associated virus (see lymphadenopathy-associated virus). The name was later changed to HIV.

Immune system: A group of specialized cells and tissues that help to defend the body against illnesses such as infections or tumors.

Immunosuppressed: The relative state of a depressed or diminished immune system resulting from use of certain medications (like cancer chemotherapy), or particular diseases (like HIV). An immunosuppressed person is more likely to get sick from infections.

Immunosuppressive drugs: A group of medications that suppress the normal function of the immune system.

Incidence: A measure of the likelihood of developing a particular condition in a given population over a specified period of time. Often measured and reported as an incidence rate.

Innate immunity: Also called inborn immunity, this term refers to a collection of cells and structures that help the body protect against foreign invaders. In distinction to the adaptive immune system, innate immunity is broader-acting (does not specifically target a given pathogen) and therefore is more blunt in its response. It is activated immediately upon exposure to a potential invader but has shorter-acting effects than those of the adaptive immune system. The innate immune system includes cells such as macrophages and natural killer cells that attack invaders in a nonspecific way.

Integrase inhibitors: A class of HIV medications that act by inhibiting the HIV integrase enzyme, a necessary step in the assembly of new HIV virions.

Kaposi's sarcoma: A type of cancer caused by human herpes virus 8 (HHV8) that results in characteristic purplish lesions on the skin. In some cases it can also affect the internal organs such as the lung, heart, and gastrointestinal tract. Kaposi's sarcoma is an AIDS-defining illness, but it can occasionally be seen in HIV-negative individuals.

Lymphadenopathy-associated virus (LAV): A once-novel retrovirus isolated from the lymph node of a patient with enlarged lymph nodes and symptoms consistent with HIV. Researchers named the virus LAV. It was later changed to HIV.

Lymphocytes: A type of white blood cell that plays an important role in the immune system. There are two main types of lymphocytes: B or T cells, which each have distinct functions in adaptive immunity (see adaptive immunity). Natural killer (NK) cells are also a type of lymphocyte that plays a role in innate immunity (see innate immunity).

Monocyte/macrophage cells: A type of white blood cell with a single large nucleus that plays a role in the immune system by "ingesting" foreign particles, invaders, debris, or dead cells. These cells are called monocytes when in your blood stream, but mature into macrophages once they have migrated into other parts of the body.

Mycobacteria: A type of infection that can cause serious disease in humans. The family mycobacteria includes many types of organisms, including the one that causes tuberculosis (*Mycobacterium tuberculosis*), leprosy (*Mycobacterium leprae*), and MAI or MAC (*Mycobacterium Avium Intracellulare* or *Mycobacterium Avium complex*), an opportunistic infection (see opportunistic infection) in patients with advanced AIDS. These organisms get their name from a waxy component (myco-) of their cell wall.

Non-nucleoside reverse transcriptase inhibitors (NNRTIs): A class of HIV medications that act by inhibiting HIV reverse transcriptase, an enzyme that is essential to the replication of HIV. These drugs bind the enzyme at a site other than its active site but still prevent its normal function.

Nucleoside reverse transcriptase inhibitors (NRTIs): A class of HIV medications that act by inhibiting HIV reverse transcriptase, an enzyme that is essential to the replication of HIV. These drugs are chemically and structurally distinct from NNRTIs (see non-nucleoside reverse transcriptase inhibitors) and inhibit replication of HIV by "looking like" building blocks used by the enzyme but preventing further elongation of the viral DNA, resulting in "chain termination." This class of drugs includes AZT (see AZT), the first medication discovered to treat HIV.

Opportunistic infection: A condition that would normally be controlled or cause limited illness in an individual with a normal immune system, but that can cause significant illness or death in someone with HIV/AIDS (or a suppressed immune system). Opportunistic infections can be caused by bacteria, viruses, mycobacteria, or fungi. They often cause illnesses that are called "AIDS-defining."

Outbreak: An increase or eruption of a particular disease in a local population that exceeds the normal background rate of this condition. Outbreaks can be epidemics (see epidemic) affecting many regions or countries or pandemics (see pandemic) affecting the world.

Pandemic: A term used to describe global disease outbreaks (see outbreak).

Parasite: An organism that lives on or in another organism (its host) and depends on it for nourishment and/or reproduction. The host typically derives no benefit and is often harmed by the parasite.

Phagocytes: A type of cell specialized in engulfing and ingesting foreign material or debris (see monocyte/macrophage cells).

Pneumocystis pneumonia: A type of opportunistic infection (see opportunistic infection) caused by a fungus that is present in the environment and causes pneumonia in persons with a suppressed immune system. The organism causing this illness was once called *Pneumocystis carinii* but has since been renamed *Pneumocystis jirovecii*. The abbreviation PCP is still used to describe pneumocystis pneumonia.

Post-exposure prophylaxis (PEP): A treatment strategy used after a high-risk exposure to try to avoid acquisition of the disease that the person exposed is at risk of developing. This strategy is used to prevent HIV, rabies, hepatitis B, and many other illnesses after exposure to them. PEP may involve use of medications, vaccines, or both—in the case of HIV it involves the use of antiretroviral medications for a limited period of time.

Prevalence: The total number of cases of a specific condition in a defined population at a given time.

Protease inhibitors: A class of HIV medications that act by inhibiting the enzyme protease, which plays an essential role in HIV replication.

Retrovirus: A group of viruses that use the enzyme reverse transcriptase to produce DNA from their RNA genome.

Reverse Transcriptase: A protein carried by HIV that allows it to convert its RNA into cDNA (see cDNA and RNA). It is the target of several drug therapies.

RNA: Ribonucleic acid (RNA), a biologic molecule similar to DNA but differing in that its nucleotides carry the sugar ribose, rather than deoxyribose—the D in DNA. Used by some viruses as genetic material, RNA is typically single-stranded, while DNA (used by humans to encode genetic material) is double-stranded. RNA can be transcribed into DNA with the help of special enzymes (as in the case of HIV replication). RNA is also used by humans as a key step in protein synthesis. DNA is transcribed into messenger RNA, which then codes for protein synthesis at cellular structures called ribosomes.

Sexually transmitted infections: A group of infections that are acquired by sexual exposure. Common examples include HIV, syphilis, gonorrhea, chlamydia, and HSV (herpes simplex virus), among others.

Simian immunodeficiency virus: The virus present in some monkeys, from which HIV is thought to be derived.

Steroids: A class of synthetic or organic compounds that includes a broad array of important molecules such as cholesterol, estradiol, testosterone, and medications such as dexamethasone or prednisone. As a class of medications, corticosteroids reduce inflammation in the body and can cause immunosuppression, especially if used at high doses or for prolonged periods of time. Anabolic steroids, a specific type of steroid, are a synthetic derivative of testosterone that use androgen receptors and are sometimes used by athletes to build muscle tissue.

Syphilis: A sexually transmitted disease caused by the spirochete *Treponema pallidum*. Syphilis characteristically causes a painless genital ulcer at its first stage and can then go on to cause rash, fever, and many other symptoms and signs affecting several parts of the body in its secondary stage. Left untreated, this illness can progress to a late tertiary stage with complications affecting the heart, blood vessels, brain, skin, and bones. After record low levels of syphilis in the United States in 2000, syphilis cases have been on the rise—especially in the men who have sex with men (MSM) group. Because syphilis and HIV share a common mechanism of transmission, and because presence of ulcerative disease increases the risk of both transmission and acquisition of HIV, special attention is focused on tracking these two epidemics (syphilis and HIV) from a public health standpoint.

T cells (or T lymphocytes): A type of lymphocyte, which is a subgroup of white blood cells, that plays a key role in adaptive immunity. T cells are subdivided into two main groups: helper T cells (or CD4 cells), which are the target of HIV infection, and cytotoxic (CD8) cells.

Toxoplasmosis: A type of opportunistic infection (see opportunistic infection) typically seen in advanced AIDS caused by a parasite called *Toxoplasma gondii*. The classic form is called cerebral toxoplasmosis and causes characteristic "ring enhancing" lesions on imaging of the brain.

Tuberculosis (TB): An infection caused by *Mycobacterium tuberculosis* that occurs worldwide but is especially prevalent in developing countries. People with suppressed immune systems, including those with HIV infection, are particularly susceptible to TB. While TB can affect any organ, it most commonly affects the lung. Left untreated, pulmonary TB can cause a severe pneumonia, fever, sweats, weight loss, coughing up blood, and ultimately death.

Varicella zoster virus (VZV): The virus responsible for chicken pox. VZV was often acquired early in life by most children. Now there is a vaccine against chicken pox and the disease is less common in childhood. After a natural exposure to varicella (i.e., chicken pox), VZV remains dormant in the body in the nervous system (in a specific area called the dorsal root ganglia). VZV can later reactivate to cause shingles or zoster, a painful vesicular rash that typically occurs on one side of the body.

Viral set point: A term that refers to the HIV viral load that is reached in early HIV infection when the virus' ability to replicate and the body's ability to hold the virus in check have reached an equilibrium. Typically ranging from a few thousand to several thousand copies of virus per ml of blood, the viral set point is believed to be predictive of disease progression. A low viral set point suggests slower disease progression, while a higher viral set point suggests more rapid disease progression.

Virus: A microscopic infectious agent that requires host cell machinery to replicate (i.e., it cannot replicate on its own). There are numerous viruses that can infect humans, including viruses causing the common cold, influenza, measles, mumps, chicken pox, hepatitis, herpes, and HIV.

Western blot: A laboratory technique used as a confirmatory test for HIV that tests for the presence of specific HIV antibodies in the blood.

Recommended Reading

Abbas, A., and A. Lichtman. 2008. *Basic Immunology.* 3rd ed. Philadelphia: Saunders, an imprint of Elsevier.

Abrams, E. J. 2000. "Opportunistic Infections and Other Clinical Manifestations of HIV Disease in Children." *Pediatric Clinics of North America* 47 (1): 79–108.

Ahmad, H., N. J. Mehta, V. M. Manikal, et al. 2001. "Pneumocystis Carinii Pneumonia in Pregnancy." *Chest* 120 (2): 666–71.

AIDSinfo, A Service of the U.S. Department of Health and Human Services. Available at: http://www.aidsinfo.nih.gov/. Accessed May 13, 2010.

Ambasa-Shisanya, C. R. 2007. "Widowhood in the Era of HIV/AIDS: A Case Study of Slaya District, Kenya." *Journal of Social Aspects of HIV/AIDS* 4 (2): 606–15.

Anderson, E., and S. Davis, eds. 2007, September 9. "AIDS Blood Scandals: What China Can Learn from the World's Mistakes." *Asia Catalyst.* Available at: http://www.asiacatalyst.org/news/AIDS_blood_scandals_rpt_0907.pdf. Accessed September 9, 2007.

Ashford, L. J. 2006, August 8. "How HIV and AIDS Affect Populations." *Population Reference Bureau.* Available at: http://www.prb.org/pdf06/HowHIVAIDSAffectsPopulations.pdf. Accessed August 25, 2008.

Augustine, J., and E. Bridges. 2008. "Young People and HIV." *Advocates for Youth.* Available at: http://www.advocatesforyouth.org/storage/advfy/documents/fshivaid.pdf. Accessed August 13, 2008.

AVERT. 2009. "HIV and AIDS in Uganda." Available at: http://www.avert.org/aids-uganda.htm. Accessed December 7, 2009.

Avert International. "History of AIDS in Africa." Available at: http://www.avert.org/history-aids-africa.htm. Accessed May 13, 2010.

Ayikukwei, Rose, D. Ngare, J. Sidle, D. Ayuku, J. Baliddawa, and J. Greene. 2008, August. "HIV/AIDS and Cultural Practices in Western Kenya: The Impact of Sexual Cleansing Rituals on Sexual Behaviours." *Culture, Health & Sexuality* 10 (6): 587–99.

Barre-Sinoussi, F., J. Chermann, F. Rey, et al. 1983. "Isolation of a T-Lymphotropic Retrovirus from a Patient at Risk for Acquired Immune Deficiency Syndrome (AIDS)." *Science* 220 (4599): 868–71.

Bartlett, J. G. 1998. "Pneumonia in the Patient with HIV Infection." *Infectious Disease Clinics of North America.* 12 (3): 807–20.

Beck, E. J., N. Mays, et al., eds. 2006. *The HIV Pandemic: Local and Global Implications.* New York: Oxford University Press.

Bell, S. K., and E. S. Rosenberg. 2009. "Case Records of the Massachusetts General Hospital: Case 11–2009: A 47-Year-Old Man with Fever, Headache, Rash, and Vomiting. *New England Journal of Medicine* 360 (15): 1540–48.

Berwick, D. 2002. "'We All Have AIDS.' Case for Reducing the Cost of HIV Drugs to Zero." *British Medical Journal* 324: 214–18.

Bollinger, R. C., S. P. Tripathy, and T. C. Quin. 1995. "The Human Immunodeficiency Virus Epidemic in India: Current Magnitude and Future Projections." *Medicine* 74 (2): 97–106.

Brau, N. 2003. "Update on Chronic Hepatitis C in HIV/HCV-Coinfected Patients: Viral Interactions and Therapy." *Journal of Acquired Immune Deficiency Syndromes* 17 (16): 2279–90.

Brenner, B., M. Roger, and L. Routy. 2007. "High Rates of Forward Transmission Events after Acute/Early HIV-1 Infection." *Journal of Infectious Diseases* 195 (7): 951–59.

Centers for Disease Control (CDC). 1981, June. "Pneumocystis Pneumonia." Available at: http://www.cdc.gov/mmwr/preview/mmwrhtml/june_5.htm. Accessed August 8, 2009.

Centers for Disease Control (CDC). 1981, July. "Kaposi's Sarcoma and Pneumocystis Pneumonia among Homosexual Men—New York City and California." Available at: http://www.aegis.com/files/mmwr/1981/MMWR04JUL81.pdf. Accessed May 13, 2010.

Centers for Disease Control (CDC). 1982. "Epidemiologic Notes and Reports Immunodeficiency among Female Sexual Partners of Males with AIDS." Available at: http://www.cdc.gov/mmwr/preview/mmwrhtml/00001221.htm. Accessed May 10, 2010.

Centers for Disease Control (CDC). 1982, July. "Opportunistic Infections and Kaposi's Sarcoma among Haitians in the United States." Available at http://www.cdc.gov/mmwr/preview/mmwrhtml/00001123.htm. Accessed May 13, 2010.

Centers for Disease Control (CDC). 1982. "Epidemiologic Notes and Reports Pneumocystis Carinii Pneumonia among Persons with Hemophilia A." Available at: http://www.cdc.gov/mmwr/preview/mmwrhtml/00001126.htm. Accessed May 13, 2010.

Centers for Disease Control (CDC). 1984. "Antibodies to a Retrovirus Etiologically Associated with Acquired Immunodeficiency Syndrome (AIDS) in Populations with Increased Incidences of the Syndrome." Available at: http://www.cdc.gov/mmwr/preview/mmwrhtml/00000368.htm. Accessed May 13, 2010.

Centers for Disease Control (CDC). 1999. "HIV and Its Transmission: HIV Prevention." Available at: http://www.cdc.gov/hiv/resources/factsheets/transmission.htm. Accessed August 13, 2008.

Centers for Disease Control (CDC). 2006. "New Estimates of U.S. HIV Prevalence, 2006 CDC HIV/AIDS Facts." Available at: http://www.cdc.gov/hiv/topics/surveillance/resources/factsheets/prevalence.htm. Accessed August 13, 2008.

Centers for Disease Control (CDC). 2007. "HIV/AIDS among Men Who Have Sex with Men." CDC HIV/AIDS Fact Sheet. Available at: http://www.cdc.gov/nchhstp/news room/docs/FastFacts-MSM-FINAL508COMP.pdf. Accessed August 16, 2008.

Centers for Disease Control (CDC). 2007. "Mother-to-Child (Perinatal) HIV Transmission and Prevention." CDC HIV/AIDS Fact Sheet. Available at: http://www.cdc.gov/hiv/topics/perinatal/resources/factsheets/perinatal.htm. Accessed August 15, 2008.

Centers for Disease Control (CDC). 2007. "The Role of STD Prevention and Treatment in HIV Prevention." CDC Fact Sheet. Available at: http://www.cdc.gov/std/hiv/STDFact-STD&HIV.htm. Accessed August 16, 2008.

Centers for Disease Control (CDC). 2008, August. "Estimates of New Infections in the United States." Available at: http://www.cdc.gov/hiv/topics/surveillance/resources/factsheets/incidence.htm. Accessed November 30, 2009.

Centers for Disease Control (CDC). 2008. "HIV/AIDS among African Americans." HIV/AIDS Fact Sheet. Available at: http://www.cdc.gov/hiv/topics/aa/resources/fact sheets/aa.htm. Accessed August 15, 2008.

Centers for Disease Control (CDC). 2008. "HIV/AIDS among Hispanics/Latinos." CDC HIV/AIDS Facts. Available at: http://www.cdc.gov/hiv/hispanics/index.htm. Accessed August 15, 2008.

Centers for Disease Control (CDC). 2008. "HIV/AIDS in the United States, National Center for HIV/AIDS, Viral Hepatitis, STD, and TB Prevention." Available at: http://www.cdc.gov/hiv/topics/surveillance/united_states.htm. Accessed August 8, 2008.

Chiappini, E., L. Galli, P. A. Tovo, et al. 2006. "Virologic, Immunologic, and Clinical Benefits from Early Combined Antiretroviral Therapy in Infants with Perinatal HIV-1 Infection." *Journal of Acquired Immune Deficiency Syndromes* 20 (2): 207–15.

Chigwedere, P., George R. Seage III, Sofia Gruskin, Ton-Hou Lee, and M. Essex. 2008. "Estimating the Lost Benefits of Antiretroviral Drug Use in South Africa." *Journal of Acquired Immune Deficiency Syndromes* 49 (4): 410–15.

CNN. 2004, November 24. "Magic Johnson Pushes HIV Awareness." Available at: http://www.cnn.com/2004/HEALTH/11/23/cnna.magic/index.html. Accessed November 9, 2009.

Cohen, D. 1992. "The Economic Impact of the HIV Epidemic." Issue Paper #2, UNDP. Available at: http://www.undp.org/hiv/publications/issues/english/issue02e.htm. Accessed November 30, 2009.

Connor, E. M., R. S. Sperling, R. Gelber, et al. 1994. "Reduction of Maternal-Infant Transmission of Human Immunodeficiency Virus Type 1 with Zidovudine Treatment." Pediatric AIDS Clinical Trials Group Protocol 076 Study Group. *New England Journal of Medicine* 331 (18): 1173–80.

Cooper, E. R., R. P. Nugent, C. Diaz, et al. 1996. "After AIDS Clinical Trial 076: The Changing Pattern of Zidovudine Use during Pregnancy, and the Subsequent Reduction in the Vertical Transmission of Human Immunodeficiency Virus in a Cohort of Infected Women and Their Infants." Women and Infants Transmission Study Group. *Journal of Infectious Diseases* 174 (6): 1207–11.

Crum, N. F., R. H. Riffenburgh, S. Wegner, et al. 2006. "Comparisons of Causes of Death and Mortality Rates among HIV-Infected Persons: Analysis of the Pre-, Early, and

Late HAART (Highly Active Antiretroviral Therapy) Eras." *Journal of Acquired Immune Deficiency Syndromes* (2):194–200.

De Cock, K. M., and H. A. Weiss. 2001. "The Global Epidemiology of HIV/AIDS." *Tropical Medicine and International Health* 5 (7): A3–A9.

De Cock, K. M., M. G. Fowler, E. Mercier, et al. 2000. "Prevention of Mother-to-Child HIV Transmission in Resource-Poor Countries: Translating Research into Policy and Practice." *Journal of the American Medical Association* 283 (9): 1175–82.

"Evolution of HIV/AIDS Prevention Programs—United States, 1981–2006." 2006. *Morbidity and Mortality Weekly Report* 55 (21): 597–603.

Fauci, A. S. 1999. "The AIDS Epidemic." *New England Journal of Medicine* 341 (14): 1046–50.

Fauci, A.S., and C. Lane. 2008. "Human Immunodeficiency Virus Disease: AIDS and Related Disorders." In *Harrison's Principles of Internal Medicine*, ed. A. S. Fauci, E. Braunwald, D. L. Kasper, et al. New York: McGraw-Hill.

Fauci, A. S., and H. C. Lane. 2008. "Chapter 182. Human Immunodeficiency Virus Disease: AIDS and Related Disorders." A. S. Fauci, E. Braunwald, D. L. Kasper, S. L. Hauser, D. L. Longo, J. L. Jameson, and J. Loscalzo. *Harrison's Principles of Internal Medicine*, 17th ed. New York: McGraw-Hill. http://accessmedicine.com/content.aspx?aid= 2904810.

Furber, A. S., I. J. Hodgson, et al. 2004. "Barriers to Better Care for People with AIDS in Developing Countries." *British Medical Journal* 329: 1281–83.

Gardner, M. B. 1996. "The History of Simian AIDS." *Journal of Medical Primatology* 25 (3):148–57.

Gilden, D. 1995. "CDC Recommends HIV Testing for All Pregnant Women." Centers for Disease Control and Prevention. *Gay Men's Health Crisis Treatment Issues* 9 (7/8): 22–23.

Gottlieb, M., R. Schroff, H. Schanker, et al. 1981. "Pneumocystis Carinii Pneumonia and Mucosal Candidiasis in Previously Healthy Homosexual Men: Evidence of a New Acquired Cellular Immunodeficiency." *New England Journal of Medicine* 305: 1425–31.

Guay, L. A., P. Musoke, T. Fleming, et al. 1999. "Intrapartum and Neonatal Single-Dose Nevirapine Compared with Zidovudine for Prevention of Mother-to-Child Transmission of HIV-1 in Kampala, Uganda: HIVNET 012 Randomised Trial." *Lancet* 354 (9181): 795–802.

"Guidelines for the Use of Antiretroviral Agents in HIV-1-Infected Adults and Adolescents." 2009. Available at: http://aidsinfo.nih.gov/contentfiles/AdultandAdolescentGL.pdf. Accessed December 3, 2009.

Hirsch, V. M., G. Dapolito, R. Goeken, and B. J. Campbell. 1995. "Phylogeny and Natural History of the Primate Lentiviruses, SIV and HIV." *Current Opinion in Genetics & Development* 5 (6): 798–806.

Hoen, B., B. Dumon, M. Harzic, et al. 1999. "Highly Active Antiretroviral Treatment Initiated Early in the Course of Symptomatic Primary HIV-1 Infection: Results of the ANRS 053 Trial." *Journal of Infectious Diseases* 180 (4): 1342–46.

Hoen, B., D. A. Cooper, F. C. Lampe, et al. 2007. "Predictors of Virological Outcome and Safety in Primary HIV Type 1-Infected Patients Initiating Quadruple Antiretroviral Therapy." QUEST GW PROB3005. *Clinical Infectious Diseases* 45 (3): 381–90.

Hollingsworth, T., R. Anderson, and C. Fraser. 2008. "HIV-1 Transmission, by Stage of Infection." *Journal of Infectious Diseases* 198 (5): 687–93.

Horne, R., V. Cooper, and M. Fisher. 2008. "Initiation of Therapy with a Subcutaneously Administered Antiretroviral in Treatment-Experienced HIV-Infected Patients: Understanding Physician and Patient Perspectives." *AIDS Care* 20 (9): 1029–38.

"I Stand with Magic." *Magic Johnson Foundation.* Available at: http://www.istandwith magic.com. Accessed August 8, 2008.

Johnson, E. 2008. "About the Foundation." *Magic Johnson Foundation.* Available at: http://www.magicjohnson.com/index.php?/foundation/aboutthefoundation/. Accessed August 12, 2008.

Johnson, W., R. Diaz, W. Flanders. 2008. "Behavioral Interventions to Reduce Risk for Sexual Transmission of HIV among Men Who Have Sex with Men." *Cochrane Database of Systematic Reviews* 3: CD001230.

Kahn, J. O., and B. D. Walker. 1998. "Acute Human Immunodeficiency Virus Type 1 Infection." *New England Journal of Medicine* 339 (1): 33–39.

Kahn, J. O., D. W. Northfelt, and S. A. Miles. 1992. "AIDS-Associated Kaposi's Sarcoma." *AIDS Clinical Reviews:* 261–80.

Kanabus, A., and J. Fredriksson. 2008, July 7. "History of AIDS." Available at: http://www.avert.org/his. Accessed August 13, 2008.

Kaplan, J. E., D. Hanson, M. S. Dworkin, et al. 2000. "Epidemiology of Human Immunodeficiency Virus-Associated Opportunistic Infections in the United States in the Era of Highly Active Antiretroviral Therapy." *Clinical Infectious Diseases* 30 Suppl 1: S5–14.

Kinloch de Loes, S., B. J. Hirschel, B. Hoen, et al. 1995. "A Controlled Trial of Zidovudine in Primary Human Immunodeficiency Virus Infection." *New England Journal of Medicine* 333 (7): 408–13.

Kitahata, M., S. Gange, and A. Abraham. 2009. "Effect of Early versus Deferred Antiretroviral Therapy for HIV on Survival." *New England Journal of Medicine* 360 (18): 1815–26.

Kovach, G. C. 2008, May 16. "Prison for Man with H.I.V. Who Spit on a Police Officer." *The New York Times.* Available at: http://www.nytimes.com/2008/05/16/us/16spit.html. Accessed August 15, 2008.

LaFraniere, Sharon. "AIDS Now Compels Africa to Challenge Widows' 'Cleansing.'" *The New York Times.* Available at: http://www.nytimes.com/2005/05/11/international/africa/11malawi.html. Accessed November 25, 2009.

Lakhashe, S., M. Thakar, S. Godbole, S. Tripathy, and R. Paranjape. 2008. "HIV Infection in India: Epidemiology, Molecular Epidemiology and Pathogenesis." *Journal of Biosciences* 33: 515–25.

Lee, S. S., Y. C. Lo, and K. H. Wong. 1996. "The First One Hundred AIDS Cases in Hong Kong." *Chinese Medical Journal* 109 (1): 70–76.

Lewis, F., G. Hughes, A. Rambaut, A. Pozniak, and A. Leigh Brown. 2008. "Episodic Sexual Transmission of HIV Revealed by Molecular Phylodynamics." *Public Library of Science Medicine* 5 (3): e50.

Libman, Howard, and Harvey Makadon. 2007. *HIV.* Philadelphia: American College of Physicians.

"Life Expectancy of Individuals on Combination Antiretroviral Therapy in High-Income Countries: A Collaborative Analysis of 14 Cohort Studies." 2008. *Lancet* 372 (9635): 293–99.

Lillo, F. B., D. Ciuffreda, F. Veglia, et al. 1999. "Viral Load and Burden Modification Following Early Antiretroviral Therapy of Primary HIV-1 Infection." Journal of *Acquired Immune Deficiency Syndromes* 13 (7): 791–96.

Lima, V. D., R. S. Hogg, P. R. Harrigan, et al. 2007. "Continued Improvement in Survival among HIV-Infected Individuals with Newer Forms of Highly Active Antiretroviral Therapy." *Journal of Acquired Immune Deficiency Syndromes* 21 (6): 685–92.

Lisziewicz, J., E. Rosenberg, J. Lieberman, et al. 1999. "Control of HIV Despite the Discontinuation of Antiretroviral Therapy." *New England Journal of Medicine* 340 (21): 1683–84.

Losina, E., B. R. Schackman, S. N. Sadownik, et al. 2009. "Racial and Sex Disparities in Life Expectancy Losses among HIV-Infected Persons in the United States: Impact of Risk Behavior, Late Initiation, and Early Discontinuation of Antiretroviral Therapy." *Clinical Infectious Diseases* 49 (10): 1570–78.

Lurie, P., and S. M. Wolfe. 1997. "Unethical Trials of Interventions to Reduce Perinatal Transmission of the Human Immunodeficiency Virus in Developing Countries." *New England Journal of Medicine* 337 (12): 853–56.

Lyles, R., A. Munoz, T. Yamashita, et al. 2000. "Natural History of Human Immunodeficiency Virus Type 1 Veremia after Seroconversion and Proximal to AIDS in a Large Cohort of Homosexual Men." *Journal of Infectious Diseases* 181: 872–80.

Malhotra, U., M. M. Berrey, Y. Huang, et al. 2000. "Effect of Combination Antiretroviral Therapy on T-Cell Immunity in Acute Human Immunodeficiency Virus Type 1 Infection." *Journal of Infectious Diseases* 181 (1): 121–31.

Malungo, J.R.S. 2001. "Sexual Cleansing (Kusalazya) and Levirate Marriage (Kunjilila mung' anda) in the Era of AIDS: Changes in Perceptions and Practices in Zambia." *Social Science & Medicine* 53: 371–82.

Markowitz, M., H. Mohri, S. Mehandru, et al. 2006. "Infection with Multidrug Resistant, Dual-Tropic HIV-1 and Rapid Progression to AIDS: A Case Report." *Lancet* 365 (9464): 1031–38.

Marks, G., N. Crepaz, and R. S. Janseen. 2006. "Estimating Sexual Transmission of HIV from Persons Aware and Unaware That They Are Infected with the Virus in the USA." *Journal Acquired Immune Deficiency Syndrome* 20 (10): 1447–50.

Masur, H., M. Michelis, J. Greene, et al. 1981. "An Outbreak of Community-Acquired Pneumocysitis Carinii Pneumonia: Initial Manifestation of Cellular Immune Dysfunction. *New England Journal of Medicine* 305: 1431–38.

Mauskopf, J. A., J. E. Paul, D. S. Wichman, A. D. White, and H. H. Tilson. 1996. "Economic Impact of Treatment of HIV-Positive Pregnant Women and Their Newborns with Zidovudine: Implications for HIV Screening." *Journal of the American Medical Association* 276 (2): 132–38.

Medina, F., L. Perez-Saleme, and J. Moreno. 2006. "Rheumatic Manifestations of Human Immunodeficiency Virus Infection." *Infectious Disease Clinics of North America* 20 (4): 891–912.

Mehandru, S., M. A. Poles, K. Tenner-Racz, et al. 2007. "Mechanisms of Gastrointestinal CD4+ T-Cell Depletion during Acute and Early Human Immunodeficiency Virus Type 1 Infection." *Journal of Virology* 81 (2): 599–612.

Mellors, J., A. Muñoz, and J. Giorgi. 1997. "Plasma Viral Load and CD4+ Lymphocytes as Prognostic Markers of HIV-1 Infection." *Annals of Internal Medicine* 126: 946–54.

Morris, K. 1998. "Short Course of AZT Halves HIV-1 Perinatal Transmission." *Lancet* 351 (9103): 651.

Murray, P., K. Rosenthal, and M. Pfaller. 2005. *Medical Microbiology.* 5th ed. Philadelphia: Elsevier Mosby.

Mwenda, K. K. 2007. "African Customary Law and Customs: Changes in the Culture of Sexual Cleansing of Widows and the Marrying of a Deceased Brother's Widow." *Gonzaga Journal of International Law* 11 (1): 1–35.

Nagappan, V., and P. Kazanjian. 2005. "Bacterial Infections in Adult HIV-Infected Patients. *HIV Clinical Trials* 6 (4): 213–28.

Oxenius, A., D. A. Price, P. J. Easterbrook, et al. 2000. "Early Highly Active Antiretroviral Therapy for Acute HIV-1 Infection Preserves Immune Function of CD8+ and CD4+ T Lymphocytes." *Procedures of the National Academy of Sciences USA* 97 (7): 3382–87.

Pandey, Arvind, Sudhir Benara, Nandini Roy, Damodar Sahu, Mariamma Thomas, Dhirenda Joshi, Utpal Sengupta, Ramesh Paranjape, Aparijita Bhalla, and Ajay Prakash. 2008. "Risk Behaviour, Sexually Transmitted Infections and HIV among Long-Distance Truck Drivers: A Cross-Sectional Survey along National Highways in India." *Journal of the Acquired Immune Deficiency Syndromes* 22 (Suppl 5): S81–S90.

Piot, P., F. Plummer, M. Rey et al. 1987. "Retrospective Seroepidemiology of AIDS Virus Infection in Nairobi Populations." *Journal of Infectious Diseases* 155 (6): 1108–12.

Poles, M. A., and D. T. Dieterich. 2000. "Hepatitis C Virus/Human Immunodeficiency Virus Coinfection: Clinical Management Issues." *Clinical Infectious Diseases* 31 (1): 154–61.

Popovic, M., M. Sarngadharan, E. Read, and R. Gallo. 1983. "Detection, Isolation, and Continuous Production of Cytopathic Retroviruses (HTLV-III) from Patients with AIDS and Pre-AIDS." *Science* 224 (4648): 497–500.

Posse, M., F. Meheus, H. van Aster, A. van der Ven, and R. Baltussen. 2008. "Barriers to Access to Antiretroviral Treatment in Developing Countries: A Review." *Tropical Medicine and International Health* 13 (7): 904–13.

Quin, M., M. Thomas, Maria Wawer, et al. 2000. "Viral Load and Heterosexual Transmission of Human Immunodeficiency Virus Type 1." *New England Journal of Medicine* 342 (13): 921–29.

"Revised Recommendations for HIV Testing of Adults, Adolescents, and Pregnant Women in Health-Care Settings." 2006. *MMWR Centers for Disease Control* 55: 1–17. Available at: http://www.cdc.gov/mmwr/preview/mmwrhtml/rr5514a1.htm. Accessed November 10, 2009.

Rosenberg, E. S., A. M. Caliendo, and B. D. Walker. 1999. "Acute HIV Infection among Patients Tested for Mononucleosis." *New England Journal of Medicine* 340 (12): 969.

Rosenberg, E. S., J. M. Billingsley, A. M. Caliendo, et al. 1997. "Vigorous HIV-1-Specific CD4+ T Cell Responses Associated with Control of Viremia." *Science* 278 (5342): 1447–50.

Rosenberg, E. S., M. Altfeld, S. H. Poon, et al. 2000. "Immune Control of HIV-1 after Early Treatment of Acute Infection." *Nature* 407 (6803): 523–26.

"Ryan's Story." Available at http://www.ryanwhite.com. Accessed August 8, 2008.

Sanders, G. D., A. M. Bayoumi, V. Sundaram, et al. 2005. "Cost-Effectiveness of Screening for HIV in the Era of Highly Active Antiretroviral Therapy." *New England Journal of Medicine* 352 (6): 570–85.

Schacker, T., A. C. Collier, J. Hughes, T. Shea, and L. Corey. 1996. "Clinical and Epidemiologic Features of Primary HIV Infection." *Annals of Internal Medicine* 125 (4): 257–64.

Schackman, B. R., K. A. Gebo, R. P. Walensky, et al. 2006. "The Lifetime Cost of Current Human Immunodeficiency Virus Care in the United States." *Medical Care* 44 (11): 990–97.

Serwadda, D., R. Mugerwa, N. Sewankambo, et al. 1985. "Slim Disease: A New Disease in Uganda and Its Association with HTLV-III Infection." *Lancet* 2 (8460): 849–52.

Shelling, G. M., ed. 2006. *AIDS Policies and Programs*. New York: Nova Science Publishers.

Shet, A., L. Berry, H. Mohri, et al. 2006. "Tracking the Prevalence of Transmitted Antiretroviral Drug-Resistant HIV-1: A Decade of Experience." *Journal of Acquired Immune Deficiency Syndromes* 41 (4): 439–46.

Shilts, R. 1987. *And the Band Played On: Politics, People and the AIDS Epidemic*. New York: St. Martin's Press.

Siegel F. P., C. Lopez, G. S. Hammer, et al. 1981. "Severe Acquired Immunodeficiency in Male Homosexuals Manifested by Chronic Perennial Ulcerative Herpes Simplex Lesions." *New England Journal of Medicine* 305: 1439–44.

Simpson, D. M. 1999. "Human Immunodeficiency Virus-Associated Dementia: Review of Pathogenesis, Prophylaxis, and Treatment Studies of Zidovudine Therapy." *Clinical Infectious Diseases* 29 (1): 19–34.

Smith, D. E., B. D. Walker, D. A. Cooper, E. S. Rosenberg, and J. M. Kaldor. 2004. "Is Antiretroviral Treatment of Primary HIV Infection Clinically Justified on the Basis of Current Evidence?" *Acquired Immune Deficiency Syndromes* 18 (5): 709–18.

Solomon, S., A. Chakraborty, and R. Yepthomi. 2004. "A Review of the HIV Epidemic in India." *AIDS Education & Prevention* 16155–169. Retrieved from Academic Search Premier database.

Steinbrook, R. 2007. "HIV in India—A Complex Epidemic." *New England Journal of Medicine* 356 (11): 1089–93.

Thisyakorn, U., M. Khongphatthanayothin, S. Sirivichayakul, et al. 2000. "Thai Red Cross Zidovudine Donation Program to Prevent Vertical Transmission of HIV: The Effect of the Modified ACTG 076 Regimen." *Acquired Immune Deficiency Syndromes* 14 (18): 2921–27.

"Treatment of HIV-1 Infected Adults with Antiretroviral Therapy." 2008. Available at: http://www.bhiva.org/TreatmentofHIV1_2008.aspx. Accessed January 10, 2010.

Trecarichi, E., M. Tumbarello, and K. Donati. 2006. "Partial Protective Effect of CCR5-Delta 32 Heterozygosity in a Cohort of Heterosexual Italian HIV-I Exposed Uninfected Individuals." *AIDS Research Therapy* 3 (22). Available at: http://www.aidsrestherapy.com/content/3/1/22. Accessed May 13, 2010.

United Nations. 2004. *The Impact of AIDS*. New York: UN Department of Economic and Social Affairs/Population Division. Available at: http://www.un.org/esa/population/publications/AIDSimpact/AIDSWebAnnounce.htm. Accessed August 25, 2008.

UNAIDS. 2008. "Report on the Global AIDS Epidemic." Available at: http://www.unaids. org/en/KnowledgeCentre/HIVData/GlobalReport/2008/. Accessed December 2009.

UNAIDS/WHO. 2007. "AIDS Epidemic Update: December 2007, UNAIDS." Available at: http://data.unaids.org/pub/EPISlides/2007/2007_epiupdate_en.pdf. Accessed August 25, 2008.

Vanhems, P., C. Lecomte, and J. Fabry. 1998. "Primary HIV-1 Infection: Diagnosis and Prognostic Impact." *AIDS Patient Care STDS* 12 (10): 751–58.

Verhoeven, D., S. Sankaran, M. Silvey, and S. Dandekar. 2008. "Antiviral Therapy during Primary Simian Immunodeficiency Virus Infection Fails to Prevent Acute Loss of CD4+ T Cells in Gut Mucosa but Enhances Their Rapid Restoration through Central Memory T Cells." *Journal of Virology* 82 (8): 4016–27.

Walensky, R. P., L. L. Wolf, R. Wood, et al. 2009. "When to Start Antiretroviral Therapy in Resource-Limited Settings." *Annals of Internal Medicine* 151 (3): 157–66.

Wawer, M., R. Gray, and N. Sweankambo. 2005. "Rates of HIV-1 Transmission per Coital Act, by Stage of HIV-1 Infection, in Rakai, Uganda." *Journal of Infectious Disease* 191 (9): 1403–9.

Weissler, J. C., and A. R. Mootz. 1990. "Pulmonary Disease in AIDS Patients." *American Journal of Medical Science* 300 (5): 330–43.

World Health Organization (WHO). 2006. "The Health of the People: The African Regional Health Report." *World Health Organization, African Regional Office*. Available at: http://www.who.int/bulletin/africanhealth/en/index.html. Accessed August 25, 2008.

Worobey, M., M. Gemmel, D. Teuwen, et al. 2008. "Direct Evidence of Extensive Diversity of HIV-1 in Kinshasa by 1960." *Nature* 455: 661–64.

Zaunders, J. J., P. H. Cunningham, A. D. Kelleher, et al. 1999. "Potent Antiretroviral Therapy of Primary Human Immunodeficiency Virus Type 1 (HIV-1) Infection: Partial Normalization of T Lymphocyte Subsets and Limited Reduction of HIV-1 DNA Despite Clearance of Plasma Viremia." *Journal of Infectious Diseases* 180 (2): 320–29.

Zolopa, A. R., and M. H. Katz. 2008. "Chapter 31: HIV Infection & AIDS." S. McPhee, M. A. Papadakis, and L. M. Tierney. *Current Medical Diagnosis & Treatment*, 50th ed. New York: McGraw-Hill. http://accessmedicine.com/content.aspx?aid=2904810.

Index

About the Authors

Sigall K. Bell, MD, is an assistant professor of medicine at Harvard Medical School in Boston, Massachusetts and the co-director of Patient Safety and Qualify Initiatives at the Institute for Professorialism and Ethical Practice, Children's Hospital Boston. She earned her medical degree from Harvard Medical School and a diploma in Tropical Medicine and Hygiene from the London School of Tropical Medicine and Hygiene. She is now on faculty in the Division of Infectious Diseases, Beth Israel Deaconess Medical Center, where she sub-specializes in HIV care, teaches medical students and trainees, and lectures nationally. Her academic focus centers on patient-doctor communication and humanism in patient care. Her work in medical education can be found the *New England Journal of Medicine*, the *New York Times*, and *Academic Medicine*.

Courtney L. McMickens, MD, MPH, is a resident physician in the department of psychiatry at the Hospital of the University of Pennsylvania. She earned her medical degree from Harvard Medical School and a master in public health degree from Harvard School of Public Health. She has conducted research on HIV/AIDS in a wide variety of academic settings, including communities in Salvador, Brazil, and Port Elizabeth, South Africa.

Kevin J. Selby, MD, is a second-year resident physician in internal medicine at the Beth Israel Deaconess Medical Center in Boston. He completed his medical doctorate at Harvard Medical School in 2009. He has conducted HIV research in Chitungwiza, Zimbabwe, focusing on mother-to-child transmission. His long-term goal is to practice primary care.